RUNNERS OF NORTH AMERICA

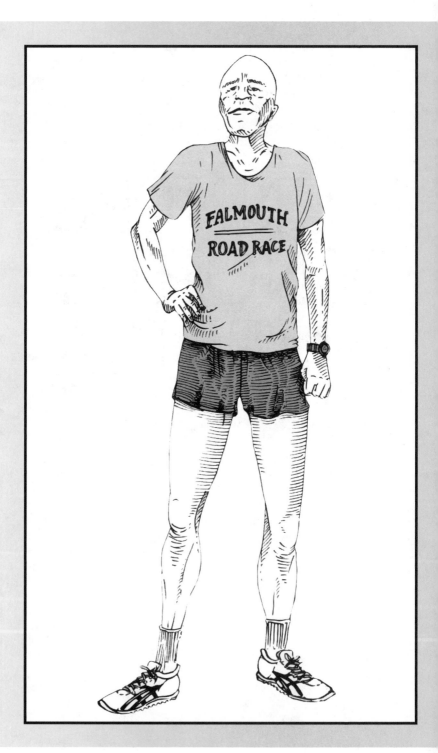

RUNNERS
OF NORTH
AMERICA

A DEFINITIVE GUIDE
TO THE SPECIES

MARK REMY

RODALE.

RODALE
wellness

Live happy. Be healthy. Get inspired.

Sign up today to get exclusive access to our authors, exclusive bonuses,
and the most authoritative, useful, and cutting edge information on health,
wellness, fitness, and living your life to the fullest.

Visit us online at RodaleWellness.com
Join us at RodaleWellness.com/Join

© 2016 by Mark Remy

All rights reserved. No part of this publication may be reproduced or transmitted in any form or by any means, electronic or mechanical, including photocopying, recording, or any other information storage and retrieval system, without the written permission of the publisher.

Rodale books may be purchased for business or promotional use or for special sales. For information, please write to:
Special Markets Department, Rodale Inc., 733 Third Avenue, New York, NY 10017

Printed in the United States of America

Rodale Inc. makes every effort to use acid-free ♾, recycled paper ♻.

Illustrations by Lucy Engleman

Image on page 105 courtesy cliparts.co

Book design by Jeff Batzli

Library of Congress Cataloging-in-Publication Data is on file with the publisher.

ISBN 978–1–62336–613–1   hardcover

Distributed to the trade by Macmillan

2   4   6   8   10   9   7   5   3   1   hardcover

RODALE.

We inspire and enable people to improve their lives and the world around them.
rodalebooks.com

To David Willey,
without whom I would
not be where I am today

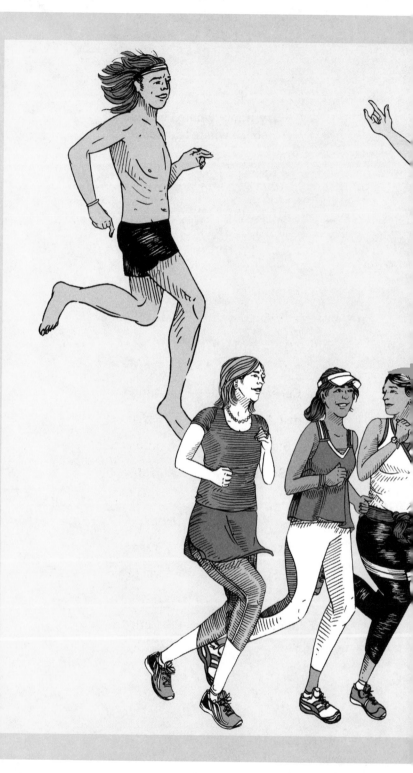

CONTENTS

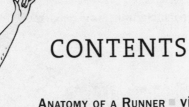

Anatomy of a Runner

From a physiological standpoint, runners are remarkably similar—though far from identical—to humans.

EXTERIOR

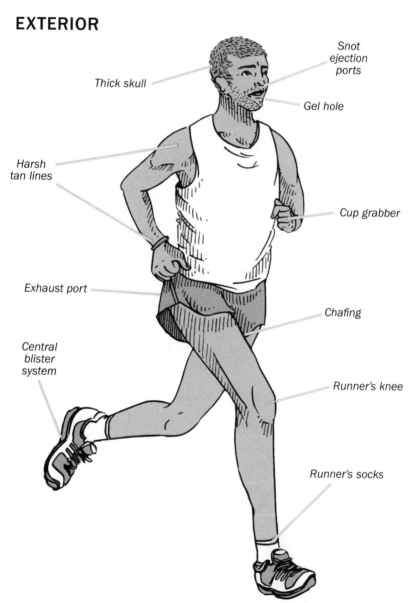

Snot ejection ports

Thick skull

Gel hole

Harsh tan lines

Cup grabber

Exhaust port

Chafing

Central blister system

Runner's knee

Runner's socks

INTERIOR

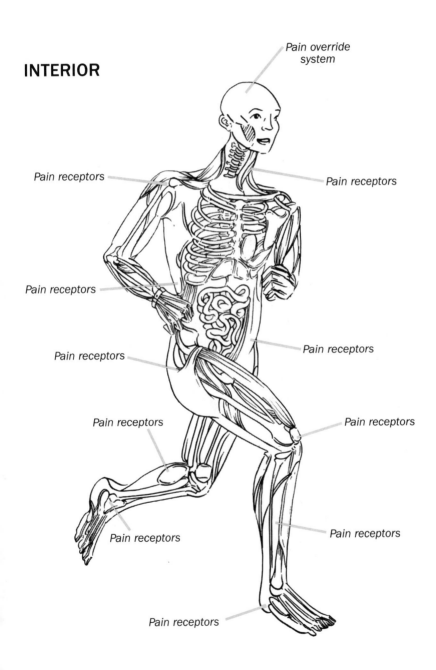

Pain override
system

Pain receptors

Pain receptors

Pain receptors

Pain receptors

Pain receptors

Pain receptors

Pain receptors

Pain receptors

Pain receptors

Pain receptors

Pain receptors

Pain receptors

INTRODUCTION

THE SUBJECT IS AN ADULT MALE. Approximately 2 meters high. Appears slightly undernourished.

He has emerged from his modest suburban nest in the early morning darkness and is standing near the street. From my vantage point in a nearby tree stand, he looks sleepy and a bit disoriented. Wearing traditional runner attire—bright-yellow, windproof jacket; black tights; gaily colored shoes—he paces, yawning. Then he freezes.

I hold my breath. Has he detected my scent? Have I spooked him?

I soon realize he is interested not in me but in his wrist. This specimen is sporting a GPS watch, a sort of ceremonial band that came into fashion among runners just in the past decade or so. Some call it "Gar-Min" and seem to worship it.

I record this in my notebook.

After a full minute and a half of staring at his wrist, the subject growls and appears agitated. He holds his wrist up, toward the stars. (Note: To appease the gods that runners believe exist in the sky, orbiting the earth?) After another minute or so, his watch beeps and he seems happy.

Suddenly another male subject comes into range, approaching the first runner. His dress and manner are similar to that of his friend. They shake hands, exchange a few inquisitive grunts, then run down the street, side by side.

As their voices and their footfalls recede into the distance, I unscrew my Thermos cap and pour myself a fresh cup of coffee. I will await their return here in my tree stand. Because it is a Sunday, that could mean waiting anywhere from 1 to 3 hours. Maybe a bit more.

When you're a runner anthropologist, it comes with the territory.

△△△△△

With their erect posture, bipedal locomotion, and vacant expressions, runners are easy to spot. Especially when they're wearing those fluorescent yellow jackets.

What's not so easy is *understanding* them. What makes these creatures tick? Can they be dangerous? And why on earth do they decorate their nipples with Band-Aids? If we humans hope to live in harmony with this burgeoning population, we must answer all these questions and more.

Since it is no longer legal to capture and experiment on them,[1] we must glean our knowledge of runners the hard way—through long, often tedious observation.

And so this is what I have done, for more than 20 years now. For most of this time, I have lived among runners, gradually earning their trust and "becoming" one of them. I ran, dressed, talked, ate, drank, and socialized like a runner. I dated other runners (before I was married). I trained and raced at distances from 5-K to the marathon. I attended mass gatherings of runners and lurked in their various online communities, watching and scribbling notes.

More than once, I ate energy "goo" from a pouch.

It has been exhilarating and exasperating, funny and sad, sweet and smelly. Mostly it has been an education. These odd creatures known as runners may seem totally alien—and in many respects they are—but they have much to teach us.

What I've learned could fill a book. And does.

My goal in writing *Runners of North America* is simple: to help you attain a better understanding of, and a deeper appreciation for, these creatures called runners—how they interact with one another (and with their environment); what they eat; how they communicate; and more.[2]

I hope you enjoy learning about runners as much as I've enjoyed studying them.

—Mark Remy, Portland, Oregon, July 2015

1 Thanks, PETA.
2 Also to make a pile of money.

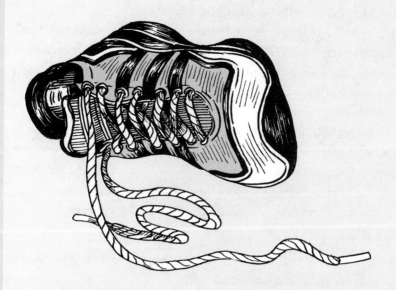

PART I

DID YOU KNOW?

Runners and humans share more than 98 percent of their DNA.

CHAPTER 1

RUNNERS: A BRIEF HISTORY

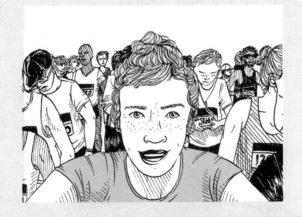

THANKS TO THE FOSSIL RECORD and early editions of Jim Fixx's *The Complete Book of Running*, we know that the species we recognize today as "runners" flourished in North America beginning circa 1977.

Back then, the landscape was much different. Hair was longer; shorts were shorter. Marathons, whose fields were thin[1] compared with today's, were still seen as exotic and strange. Women were rarely spotted running in public. And Starbucks had not yet expanded beyond its single store in Seattle to bring its clean public restrooms to every city from coast to coast.[2]

Most notably, runners themselves were much more rare. While today's runners may be considered oddballs, the runners of yesteryear were seen as downright crazy, when they were seen at all. The runners of today owe a debt of gratitude to these early pioneers, who made it seem okay to venture onto public roads wearing what is essentially underwear and to bounce up and down while waiting to cross the street.

While their dress and hairstyles differed greatly, in certain other ways the earliest runners bore an uncanny resemblance to the runners of today—they were often lean and hungry-looking, wore unusual footwear, and sometimes identified themselves by wearing numbers on their chests.[3]

> ### Runner Relic
>
> #### *The Terrycloth Headband*
>
> *In addition to their long hair and sideburns, early runners often boasted lush terrycloth headbands. Over time these accessories, which conferred no real competitive or evolutionary advantage, atrophied and disappeared. You might see a smaller, vestigial headband today, but nearly always it is part of a costume or a self-conscious "throwback" to an earlier era. The last sincerely worn headband in the wild was seen in 1984.*

---

1 In at least two senses of the word.

2 Where did runners use the bathroom before Starbucks came along? No one knows.

3 Well, not on their chests. I mean on the front of their shirts.

Runners are very closely related to humans, at least physiologically, as this chart demonstrates:

	RUNNER	HUMAN
PRIMATE?	YES	YES
OPPOSABLE THUMBS?	YES	YES
USE TOOLS?	YES	YES
NURSE THEIR YOUNG?	YES	YES
TALK ABOUT THEIR "SPLITS"?	YES	NO
SLEEP IN ON SUNDAY MORNINGS?	NO	YES
CALL RUNNING SHOES "SNEAKERS"?	NO	YES
MATE FOR LIFE?	NO	NO

Q&A

Q: *My father, who ran marathons as a young man in the 1970s, has told me that at his peak he ran in the 2:45 to 2:50 range and that he routinely finished in the middle of the pack! Is he suffering from the early stages of dementia?* —**Nick, Fort Wayne, Indiana**

A: *No! Well, maybe he is. But his marathoning anecdotes aren't evidence of it. In the 1960s and '70s road racing was much more competitive. By definition, anyone who entered a marathon back then was a Serious Runner, interested not only in bettering his own personal-best time but also in beating those around him. (Back then, marathon-running was virtually a male-only endeavor.) Today, with marathon fields much larger and much slower (on average), a 2:45 may well get you a top 10 finish, depending on the size of the race. This causes Serious Runners (page 32) no end of grief.*

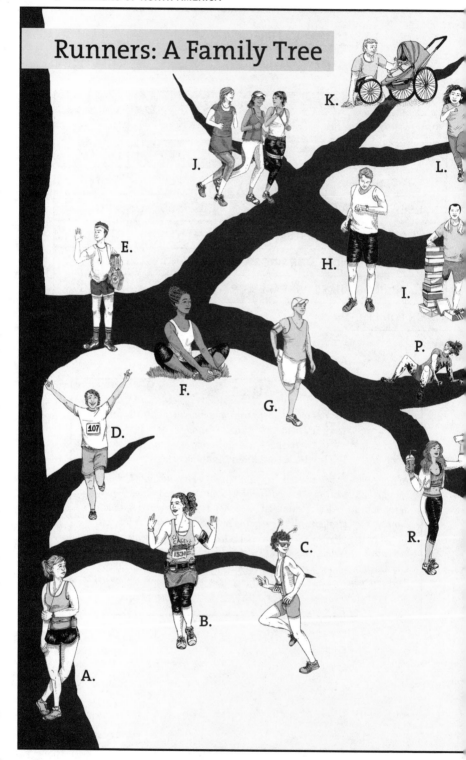

Runners: A Family Tree

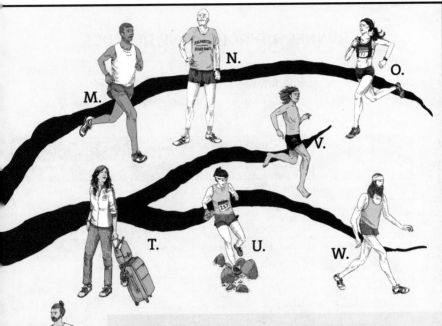

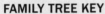

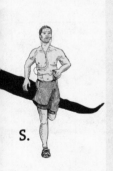

FAMILY TREE KEY

A. The Newbie
(Lopus novus) See page 12

B. The Charity Runner
(Lopus altruistus) See page 65

C. The Weirdo Runner
(Lopus prepostus) See page 26

D. The Bucket Lister
(Lopus yolo) See page 24

E. The Club Runner
(Lopus socialis) See page 18

F. The "I'm Not a Real Runner" Runner
(Lopus modestus) See page 15

G. The Dramatic Weight Loss Runner
(Lopus saladus) See page 45

H. The 7:00-Minute-Mile Guy
(Lopus mono velocitus) See page 59

I. The Gear Addict
(Lopus productus) See page 62

J. The Mom Runner
(Lopus matercula) See page 51

K. The Dad Runner
(Lopus paternus) See page 54

L. The Kid Runner
(Lopus juvenilis) See page 76

M. The Serious Runner
(Lopus fastholus) See page 32

N. The Grizzled Vet
(Lopus veteranus) See page 56

O. The Elite Runner
(Lopus elitus) See page 36

P. The Adventure Racer
(Lopus adrenalinus) See page 42

Q. The High-Intensity Cross-Trainer
(Lopus explosivus) See page 39

R. The Fashion Mag Runner
(Lopus lulemonus) See page 29

S. The Fitness Runner
(Lopus vanitus) See page 21

T. The Serial Marathoner
(Lopus pheidippidus) See page 67

U. The Ultra Runner
(Lopus extremus) See page 73

V. The Barefoot Runner
(Lopus naturalis) See page 48

W. The Trail Runner
(Lopus granolus) See page 70

RUNNERS THROUGH THE DECADES

The North American runner has evolved over the years, adapting to changes in his environment, including new threats, technologies, food sources, and fashion—even to changes seen in other runners. Here is an overview.

	FASHION	TECHNOLOGY	DIET	HAIR	QUIRKS	PHYSIOLOGY OF AVERAGE SPECIMEN
1950s	Baggy shorts and simple leather shoes	Analog stopwatch held by man wearing fedora and wool trousers	Meat and potatoes	Crew cuts or Brylcreem-assisted styles; no facial hair	Says things like "gee" and "swell"	Lean, strong
1960s	Short shorts; cotton tees or tank tops; canvas sneakers; gray sweats	Wristwatch	Grains and vegetables; pasta; brown rice	Longer and bushier, including facial hair	Thinks a woman's uterus will fall out if she runs a marathon	Lean, strong
1970s	Shorter shorts; brand-name running shoes made of synthetic materials; tube socks; headbands	Simple digital watch; pedometer	Granola; wheat germ; yogurt	Moderately long, sometimes feathered; remarkable mustaches	May call self "jogger" and be okay with that	Mostly lean, pretty strong
1980s	"Sweat suits"; matching "jogging" outfits	More advanced digital watch; Sony Walkman	Lean Cuisine; fat-free cookies; salt tablets	Ample and hair-spray-hardened or permed	Time spent drying hair postrun often surpasses time spent running	Average
1990s	Nylon "tracksuits"; polyester running shorts; bright colors	Even more advanced digital watch; Breathe Right strip across nose	Sports drinks; energy bars; primitive energy gels; lots of pasta	Lower volume; possibly gelled or moussed	Believes that stuffing self silly with spaghetti will lead to better marathon times	Pretty average
2000s	"Technical" tees; nylon shorts; FuelBelt	iPod; GPS watch	Sports drinks; energy bars; advanced energy gels; more pasta	Lower volume; little to no gel or mousse	May be seen wearing FuelBelt even in a 5-K	Some extra padding
2010s	Compression socks; even more "technical" clothing	Activity-tracking bracelet; iPod; smartphone	Dozens of new sports drinks, energy bars, and gels; "ancient grains"; meat; gluten-free crackers	Short, unremarkable	Often pays to run in crowded races, then isolates self with earbuds or headphones	Extra padding

Uniquely among known species, runners evolve on a macro and micro level—that is, runners as a group evolve over decades, while an individual runner may himself evolve over the course of his life. This evolution may occur even down to the supermicro level—for instance, a runner's feet may evolve over the course of her running life, from smooth and attractive to gnarled and calloused.

It is thought that the progenitor of all North American runners was likely a farmer or laborer who migrated to the continent from Europe, crossing the Atlantic in the cargo hold of a steamship in search of free bagels.

Today runners can be found on all seven continents, in habitats ranging from cramped urban settings to sprawling rural countryside.

THE EVOLUTION OF RUNNING SHOES—A TIMELINE

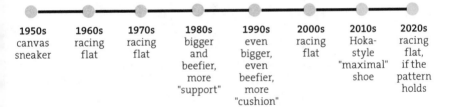

1950s	1960s	1970s	1980s	1990s	2000s	2010s	2020s
canvas sneaker	racing flat	racing flat	bigger and beefier, more "support"	even bigger, even beefier, more "cushion"	racing flat	Hoka-style "maximal" shoe	racing flat, if the pattern holds

Barefoot Runners

No discussion of the evolution of runners would be complete without a mention of the "barefoot running" phenomenon.

DID YOU KNOW?

Scientists believe there are as many as a dozen as-yet-undiscovered subspecies of runners in remote regions of the world, such as the Amazon basin and Nebraska.

CHAPTER 2

THE 23 SUBSPECIES OF RUNNERS

BY DEFINITION, ALL RUNNERS SHARE certain common characteristics—namely, a seemingly hardwired desire to run and to talk about running, and an insatiable appetite for free bagels and bananas. Beyond these superficial commonalities, however, runners are a remarkably diverse species. Researchers have identified no fewer than 23 subspecies of runners, and while the layperson may find them indistinguishable, each has its own physiological adaptations and psychosocial quirks.

Let's take a closer look.

The Newbie
Lopus novus

All runners begin as the common, unassuming creature known as the Newbie. Over time the Newbie will grow up and out of the subspecies, evolving gradually into another, more specialized subspecies, from Fitness Runner to Mom Runner or Trail Runner to Serial Marathoner. Even Serious Runners and Elites begin their running lives as Newbies.

However, not all Newbies "make it" and become full-fledged runners. For a variety of reasons, a Newbie may decide that running is not for her. And so her running life will end, just as it was beginning, and she will find another species to identify with.

Think of the Newbie, in these instances, as a caterpillar who becomes not a butterfly but a mountain biker. Such is the miracle of nature.

By definition the Newbie is new to running and therefore tends to be extremely self-conscious. This can be a good thing—i.e., insofar as it keeps the Newbie humble and encourages her to take things easy—but those Newbies who lack the capacity to harness these feelings and ultimately rein them in may soon find themselves giving up. Fortunately, this is the exception and not the rule.

☐ **Distinguishing characteristics:** The Newbie is marked by his tentative gait, his tentative demeanor, and his tentative way of asking tentative questions. This is a positive trait with clear evolutionary advantages.[1]

---

1 Those few Newbies who display absolute confidence in their running—how they do it, how often, how fast, in what shoes, etc.—have a habit of morphing suddenly from Newbie to Injured Runner, and then from Injured Runner to Former Runner.

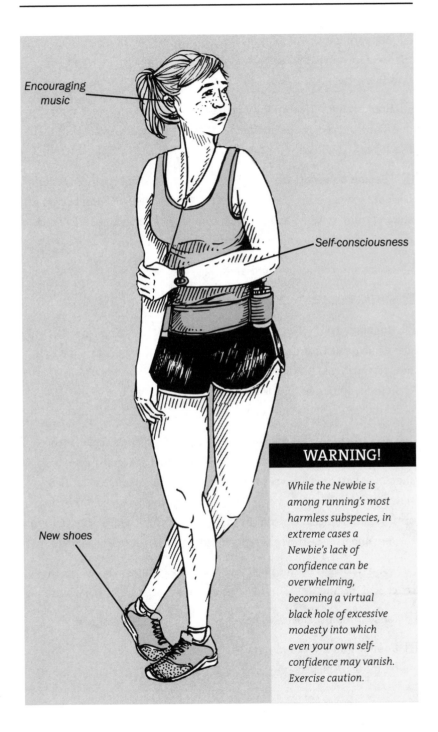

Encouraging music

Self-consciousness

New shoes

WARNING!

While the Newbie is among running's most harmless subspecies, in extreme cases a Newbie's lack of confidence can be overwhelming, becoming a virtual black hole of excessive modesty into which even your own self-confidence may vanish. Exercise caution.

☐ **Appearance:** The Newbie looks less like a "runner" and more like "a regular person who has bought some running shoes and isn't entirely sure how to use them."

☐ **Habitat:** Specialty running stores, where she is asking lots of (tentative) questions and apologizing for them; suburban sidewalks, early in the morning or late at night, where she does most of her runs, so as not to be seen

☐ **Feeding behavior:** The Newbie tends to eat well, not because he always has but because he has just subscribed to *Runner's World* and/or bought a stack of running books and therefore suddenly has an abundance of recipes for beet smoothies and butternut squash soup.

☐ **Sounds:** Panting. But *happy* panting.

☐ **Mating call:** "Am I doing this right?"

☐ **Running style:** You guessed it—tentative. The Newbie employs an easily identifiable shuffling gait, with shoulders hunched slightly forward as if he is trying to make himself as small and inconspicuous as possible. Over time, as his spine develops, the Newbie's running style will evolve as well, becoming more upright and open.

When running with others, especially in races, the Newbie will often employ another style of running—a sort of "sprint/sag" strategy wherein she surges past her fellow runners, head down and arms pumping, before slowing to a near-crawl. Once recovered, the Newbie will repeat this process until she is no longer able to sprint, at which point she will shuffle along for the remainder of the run or race or just go get an iced coffee or something.

Again, over time this habit will diminish as the Newbie learns the concept of "pacing."

☐ **Closest relatives:** The Kid Runner; the "I'm Not a Real Runner" Runner

☐ **Enemies and threats:** His or her own sense of self-doubt; doing "too much, too fast"; blisters

The "I'm Not a Real Runner" Runner

Lopus modestus

Possibly the most common of all runner subspecies, the "I'm Not a Real Runner" (INARR) Runner is marked by a sense of humility that can range from mild to crippling. Curiously, things like mileage (per run, per week, lifetime), pace, and even number of races under his belt have no influence on the demeanor of the INARR Runner. Whether he runs 5 miles a week or 50, the "I'm Not a Real Runner" Runner will maintain during conversations with others—and especially with other running enthusiasts that he considers "real"—that he is Not a Real Runner.

☐ **Distinguishing characteristics:** Self-deprecation; reluctance to talk about his or her own running habits; nonflashy running shoes and attire

☐ **Appearance:** Meek

☐ **Habitat:** *Lopus modestus* can be found just about anywhere runners have a presence. Usually standing quietly in a corner.

☐ **Feeding behavior:** Most INARR Runners eat quite "normally" (i.e., in a way that humans would find familiar), though a few can be surprisingly austere in their eating habits. Researchers speculate that this occurs in the meekest of the meek INARR Runners, as their lack of self-worth creeps into even their diet—i.e., they feel that because they aren't real runners, they haven't earned the right to indulge in such things as 2% milk for their coffee or a second helping of watercress.

☐ **Sounds:** "I'm not a real runner. I just do a few miles, a few times a week. Nothing serious."

☐ **Mating call:** "See? Now, you're a *real* runner."

☐ **Running style:** Paradoxically, most INARR Runners run quite a bit. Even if they don't run very far—and, again, some of them do—they run very consistently. The INARR typically employs an efficient, businesslike running form, head down and arms close to the torso in a manner that says, "Pay no attention to me. I am not a real runner."

☐ **Closest relatives:** The Bucket Lister; the Mom Runner; the Charity Runner

☐ **Enemies and threats:** The Serious Runner; the Trail Runner; the Ultra Runner; the Barefoot Runner; the Grizzled Vet; the congratulatory postrace pat on the back, which may serve to reinforce the INARR's feeling that he is a total fraud

WARNING!

While they may seem endearing at first, the protestations of the INARR Runner can quickly grow tiresome. You may be tempted, after the third or fourth instance of vocal self-abasement, to shake the specimen by the shoulders and shout, "You are so a runner! You run! For cripe's sake!" This may panic him or her. And even a timid creature like Lopus modestus, *when panicked, can scratch and bite.[2]*

---

2 *It is rare, but some* Lopus modestus *in a sudden fight-or-flight situation may vomit on you as a means of defending themselves.*

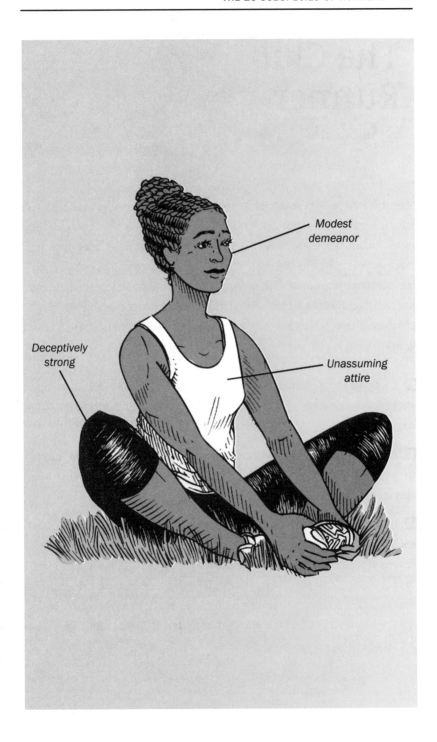

The Club Runner

Lopus socialis

The Club Runner is motivated less by inward things like physical health, weight loss, or fitness goals and more by the social aspect of running—very much including the happy hour drinks following every Thursday evening's track workout. For this reason, the Club Runner is always a member of at least one running group, club, or organization, whether formal or informal, and is naturally drawn to others who similarly value camaraderie and companionship. If the Club Runner couldn't run with others, she likely wouldn't run at all.

☐ **Distinguishing characteristics:** Wide smile; car plastered with bumper stickers from local running club(s); often seen carrying a cooler and a large bag of ice

☐ **Appearance:** Remarkably unremarkable. Most Club Runners look like they could live next door to you. Which they might. Don't worry—this sub-species of runners is one of the friendliest.

☐ **Habitat:** By definition, most Club Runners live in towns and cities large enough to have running clubs (and good bars)—or, at a minimum, casual groups of runners that morph into their own "clubs." Club Runners are easy to spot at your local supermarket; they'll be the ones wearing running shoes and T-shirts for your town's annual half-marathon while buying hot dogs, buns, and beer for the BBQ after their club's upcoming five-dollar 5-K race.

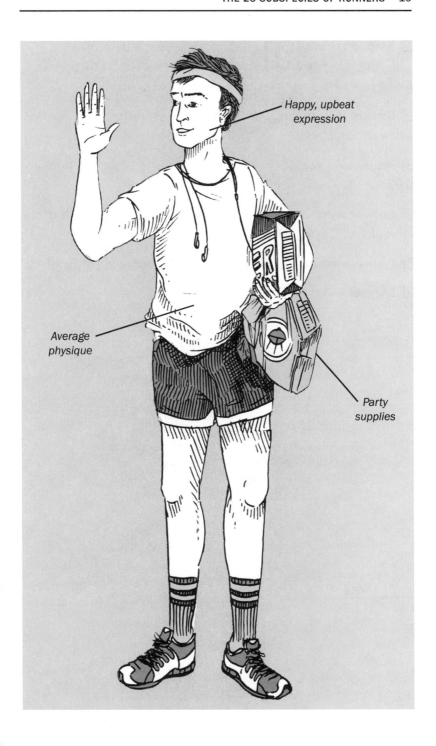

☐ **Feeding behavior:** Club Runners consume most of their calories at potluck dinners following local club-sponsored races and at happy hour get-togethers following the club's weekly track workouts.

☐ **Sounds:** Laughter; inside jokes cultivated over hundreds of miles with fellow Club Runners

☐ **Mating call:** "Hey, we do a weekly long run every Sunday, leaving from the bakery. You should join us."

☐ **Running style:** Loose and casual; typically side by side with at least one other Club Runner, to facilitate discussion

☐ **Closest relatives:** The "I'm Not a Real Runner" Runner; the Grizzled Vet

☐ **Enemies and threats:** The Serious Runner

WARNING!

Use caution when socializing with a Club Runner. Due to their experience at club events, many Club Runners have an astonishing tolerance for alcohol and can lead others to overindulge as they try to keep up. In extreme cases, this can lead to registering for marathons while drunk.

The Fitness Runner

Lopus vanitus

Most, if not all, runners share a desire to be fit. For the Fitness Runner, how-ever, that is where motivation begins and ends. He is running with the express intent of attaining fitness. Period. If the Fitness Runner could take a pill that would deliver all the benefits of running, he would. But no such pill exists. He knows, because he is at GNC at least once a week and he would have seen it by now.

Note: It is not by accident that I am using the pronouns "he" and "his" in this description. The Fitness Runner is almost exclusively male. (There is no direct female analogue, though the Fashion Mag Runner comes close.)

☐ **Distinguishing characteristics:** Earbuds; various electronic devices in hand(s); terrific hair; look of vague discomfort; jogs in place at intersections

☐ **Appearance:** Baggy shorts, with or without compression shorts under-neath; developed arms, chest, and shoulders; the kind of calves you do not get from running; suspiciously clean running shoes

☐ **Habitat:** Public paths and trails; gym treadmills. When not running, the Fitness Runner may be found "shooting hoops" or "lifting."

☐ **Feeding behavior:** Lots of protein

☐ **Sounds:** "Time for cardio"

☐ **Mating call:** "Time for cardio"

☐ **Running style:** Long strides. Upper body appears stiff and tense, mostly due to the fact that the Fitness Runner, while running, is also flexing most of his muscles. Some Fitness Runners may display a running form that goes beyond "stiff and tense" to outright "ungainly"—jerking their arms and shoulders, for instance, almost violently back and forth while their feet slap the ground hard with each stride. It will appear as if their very bodies are rebelling against the act of running. Which they may well be. Still, they grind on. This is the ethos of the Fitness Runner.

☐ **Closest relatives:** The Mom Runner; the Dad Runner; the Fashion Mag Runner

☐ **Enemies and threats:** The Serious Runner; the Trail Runner; the Ultra Runner; the Barefoot Runner; the Grizzled Vet

WARNING!

Many Fitness Runners stretch before they run, using techniques that border on violent. These stretches are so poorly conceived and executed, in fact, that there have been a few recorded instances of bystanders injuring their groins just by watching them.

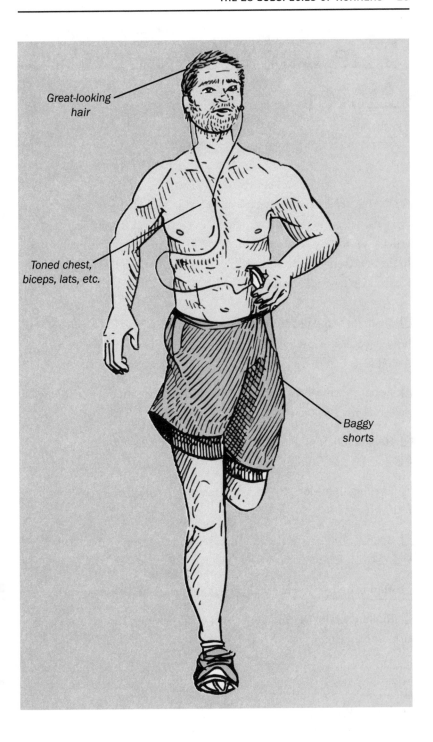

Great-looking
hair

Toned chest,
biceps, lats, etc.

Baggy
shorts

The Bucket Lister

Lopus yolo

For the Bucket Lister, running is a means to an end. That "end" is a literal one—namely, a marathon finish line. Once he reaches it, the Bucket Lister will pause[3] to cross "run a marathon" off his bucket list before moving on to the next item, which will possibly be "run with the bulls," if his bucket list is in alphabetical order.

☐ **Distinguishing characteristics:** New running shoes; scar from bungee jumping accident; desire to Get the Most Out of Life and to Live Each Day As If It's His Last

☐ **Appearance:** Happy; reasonably fit; at least one tattoo, because why not, You Only Live Once

☐ **Habitat:** Comfortable middle-class neighborhoods; tattoo parlors; the gym

☐ **Feeding behavior:** The Bucket Lister will try anything once. Even rattlesnake![4]

☐ **Sounds:** "Let's do this!"; "Did I ever tell you about my trip to Machu Picchu?"

☐ **Mating call:** "Life is short. Let's get another pitcher of margaritas."

☐ **Running style:** The Bucket Lister runs the way he does everything else—with gusto.

---

3 *Figuratively, we hope. Otherwise he will risk causing a pileup as exhausted runners bump into him.*
4 *During a backpacking trip in Thailand.*

☐ **Closest relatives:** The Club Runner; the Mom Runner; the Dad Runner

☐ **Enemies and threats:** The Serious Runner; the Trail Runner; the Ultra Runner; the Barefoot Runner; the Grizzled Vet

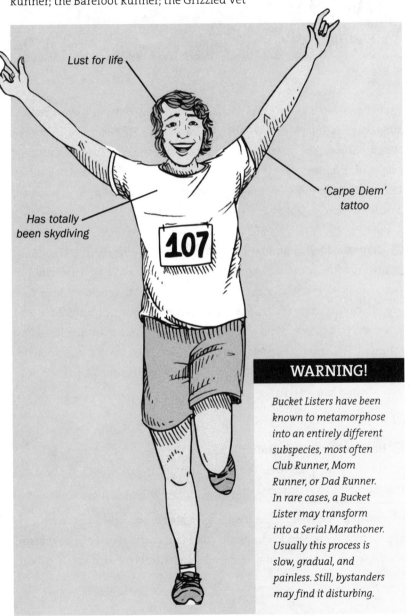

Lust for life

'Carpe Diem' tattoo

Has totally been skydiving

107

WARNING!

Bucket Listers have been known to metamorphose into an entirely different subspecies, most often Club Runner, Mom Runner, or Dad Runner. In rare cases, a Bucket Lister may transform into a Serial Marathoner. Usually this process is slow, gradual, and painless. Still, bystanders may find it disturbing.

The Weirdo Runner

Lopus prepostus

Far out on the fringes of runnerdom, often wearing comically oversized sunglasses, rainbow wigs, and/or a springy "antenna" headband, lives the Weirdo Runner. The rarest of runner subspecies, the Weirdo plays a crucial role in running's ecosystem, keeping things "fun" in a sport that can suffer from overearnestness and making other runners seem somewhat normal by comparison.

☐ **Distinguishing characteristics:** Where should we start? The Weirdo Runner is nothing *but* distinguishing characteristics. They vary wildly from one specimen to another, however, so it's hard to generalize here. One Weirdo Runner may run in a Speedo. Another, face paint or cutoff blue jeans with old canvas sneakers. The point is, each Weirdo Runner has a "thing," a trademark that gets him noticed (e.g., "Hey, there's that guy who races in a tutu"). The one constant is that the overall impression is one of weirdness.

☐ **Appearance:** Weird

☐ **Habitat:** The Weirdo Runner is all over the map—both in terms of quirks and of geography. He or she can be found in just about any climate that's hospitable to runners. Usually on the fringes.

☐ **Feeding behavior:** While it may seem at odds with their outward appearance, most Weirdo Runners enjoy a fairly normal diet of lean protein, grains, fruits, vegetables, and whatever small insects they can catch and eat.

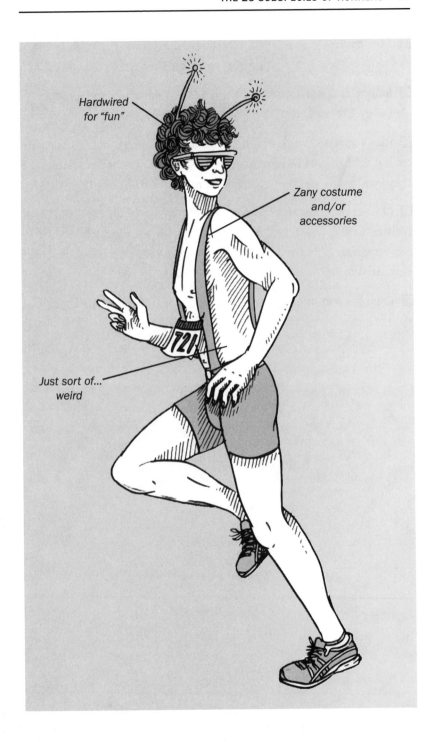

☐ **Sounds:** Tinny music—typically something like jazz fusion, rockabilly, or '80s New Wave—emanating from small speakers worn on their person

☐ **Mating call:** Unknown. It is believed that Weirdo Runners reproduce asexually, like water fleas and aphids.

☐ **Running style:** The technical nature of the Weirdo's running style varies, but the hallmark is one of pure joy. Weirdo Runners may be weird, but they love to run and they have a ball doing it. "Bopping" may be involved.

☐ **Closest relatives:** Strangely enough, the Weirdo Runner's closest relative is the Grizzled Vet. Both subspecies share a distinct lack of self-consciousness. In fact, many Weirdo Runners, over time, evolve to become Grizzled Vets.

☐ **Enemies and threats:** None, because no one feels threatened by the Weirdo Runner

WARNING!

Despite their seeming confidence, Weirdo Runners tend to be very sensitive. It is not advised to call a Weirdo Runner "weird," even if you mean it as a compliment, which you probably do.

The Fashion Mag Runner

Lopus lulemonus

With her matching sports bra ($54), tech racerback shirt ($48), and crop pants with mesh panels and flat seams in four-way Lycra stretch fabric ($96), the Fashion Mag Runner looks *terrific*. She runs "a couple times a week," but most days spends several hours dressed like she's about to go for a run.

☐ **Distinguishing characteristics:** Bright plumage and snug garments that highlight and accentuate the hips, bust, and tummy; earbuds plugged into hot-pink or lime-green iPod Nano; smoothie

☐ **Appearance:** Full makeup, regardless of weather or time of day; high, neat ponytail; at least one small, tasteful tattoo or body piercing; annoyingly fit

☐ **Habitat:** High-end athletic apparel shops; Starbucks; on the treadmill at your gym, with a copy of *Elle*

☐ **Feeding behavior:** Most Fashion Mag Runners, because they read fashion magazines, love to read recipes for couscous salads and chia seed smoothies while they eat gravy fries.

☐ **Sounds:** "I love your top."

☐ **Mating call:** Fashion Mag Runners don't need mating calls.

☐ **Running style:** Bouncy; tall; relaxed shoulders; short strides; eyes downward, fixed on phone

☐ **Closest relatives:** The Mom Runner; the Bucket Lister; the Charity Runner; the High-Intensity Cross-Trainer

☐ **Enemies and threats:** The Serious Runner; the Trail Runner; the Ultra Runner; the Barefoot Runner; the Grizzled Vet; lampposts, potholes, and other things she might run into while looking at her phone

WARNING!

The Fashion Mag Runner will almost certainly cause you to question your own fashion choices. This may lead you to question every other choice you have made, as you imagine her life, the rest of which is probably just as perfect as her appearance, which may lead to depression. Also, the Fashion Mag Runner tends to be highly attractive. This may be hazardous for bystanders whose wives catch them staring.

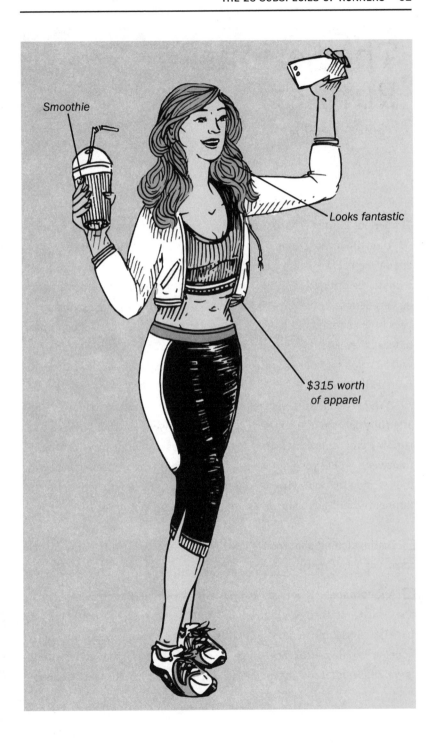

The Serious Runner

Lopus fastholus

The Serious Runner is hard to pin down, and not just because he is so fast. (Historically, most Serious Runners have been male, though this has changed quickly; it's rare but not unheard of for a pair of Serious Runners to mate, resulting in offspring that, in theory at least, have the potential to be *Very* Serious Runners.) Many Serious Runners are enigmas, giving up very little about themselves or what motivates them to run as much, or as hard, as they do. All you know for sure about the Serious Runner is that he will beat you soundly in a race of nearly any distance. Probably without even really trying.

While Serious Runners are born Serious, many—though certainly not all—fully develop in their late teens and early twenties, through collegiate running programs. Others may not achieve peak Seriousness until their midtwenties or beyond; in these cases, the subject may in fact have begun life as, say, a Serious Swimmer or Serious Cyclist and become a Serious Runner through a gradual and sometimes painful mutation.

☐ **Distinguishing characteristics:** Lanky frame; thin arms; team uniform; vaguely unnerving eyes

☐ **Appearance:** It is impossible to describe the Serious Runner without using the word *gaunt*. Their height may vary from "sort of short" to "pretty tall," but all Serious Runners share a reedlike physique, sunken cheeks, and hip bones you could use to crack an egg. Also, it may look as if the Serious Runner is walking around sucking in his gut. He's not. That's just the way he looks.

Upon very close inspection, the Serious Runner may appear to be vibrating.

Paradoxically, some Serious Runners may actually look relaxed and completely at ease as they shamble around, smiling, quick to laugh, in no particular hurry to be anywhere. This is the demeanor of someone with absolute confidence. Specifically the absolute confidence that their marathon pace would leave you dry-heaving onto your shoes if you tried to maintain it even for a few hundred meters.

☐ **Habitat:** On the road, running. Twice a day, at least. When they aren't running, Serious Runners enjoy napping, foam rolling, and staring straight ahead as they hold their palms over an open flame. Also, some Serious Runners find work at Serious Running Stores, where they pace the floor with nervous energy, waiting for someone to come in and say the need some new "tennis shoes."

☐ **Feeding behavior:** They'll eat little before or during a race, but otherwise Serious Runners are capable of consuming impressive amounts of food, given their lack of gut. This is not to say that they take advantage of this capability. With few exceptions, they do not. Instead they eat quietly and judiciously, if not sparingly, and make sure everyone knows it when they *do* enjoy a large meal—especially if that large meal involves something "bad" for them, e.g., a bacon cheeseburger with a fried egg on top.

☐ **Sounds:** The Serious Runner is a man of few words, even if she is in fact a woman. These words include:

Job—short for, "Good job," uttered to a fellow competitor after a race or, more rarely, a workout. Usually accompanied by a businesslike hand slap, fist bump, high five, and/or a curt nod of the head.

And . . . Actually, that's about it.

You rarely if ever hear a Serious Runner making sounds while racing, because those sounds could telegraph weakness, and weakness is for the weak. Which is a phrase the Serious Runner may or may not have tattooed on his ankle, in Chinese characters.

☐ **Mating call:** "Job."

☐ **Running style:** Loose; graceful; relaxed

☐ **Closest relatives:** The Grizzled Vet

☐ **Enemies and threats:** The Bucket Lister; the Mom Runner; the Charity Runner

---

WARNING!

Looking a Serious Runner directly in the eye may cause unease or discomfort. Mostly because you may get the feeling that the Serious Runner is judging you and/or wondering how much effort it would take to crush you, either in a race or literally.[5] Never approach an injured Serious Runner. An injured Serious Runner has not been running lately and is therefore extremely dangerous.

---

5 You may get this feeling because that is EXACTLY what the Serious Runner is thinking.

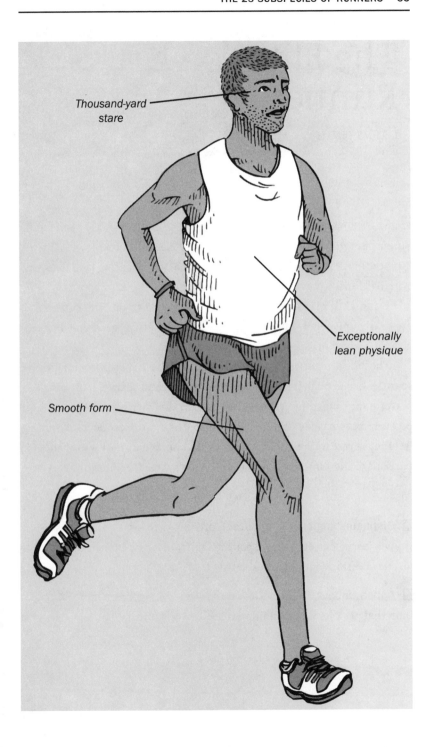

Thousand-yard stare

Exceptionally lean physique

Smooth form

The Elite Runner
Lopus elitus

From a distance, the Elite Runner may look a lot like just another Serious Runner. But make no mistake—Elites are in a class all of their own. Elite Runners make Serious Runners look like sweat suit–wearing mall walkers with bad hips.

Not that this is their intention. Far from it. As a group, Elite Runners are nearly universally humble and polite. They're just so good that anyone else can't help but seem clumsy and slow by comparison.

The Elite Runner, tragically, has a comparatively short running lifespan. He or she might expect anywhere from 5 to 10 years of truly peak performance, meaning "years in which he or she can realistically vie for podium spots, paydays, and sponsorships." There are exceptions, of course. But they're rare. Perhaps it is this relatively brief window—inviting comparisons to shooting stars and the like—that makes the Elite Runner seem so special.

☐ **Distinguishing characteristics:** Matching shoes and clothing—shorts, singlet, jacket, hat, etc.—from sponsor; faint aura of awesomeness that's visible in certain lighting conditions

☐ **Appearance:** Always shorter and smaller than you'd imagined. Other than that, they look quite similar to the Serious Runner.

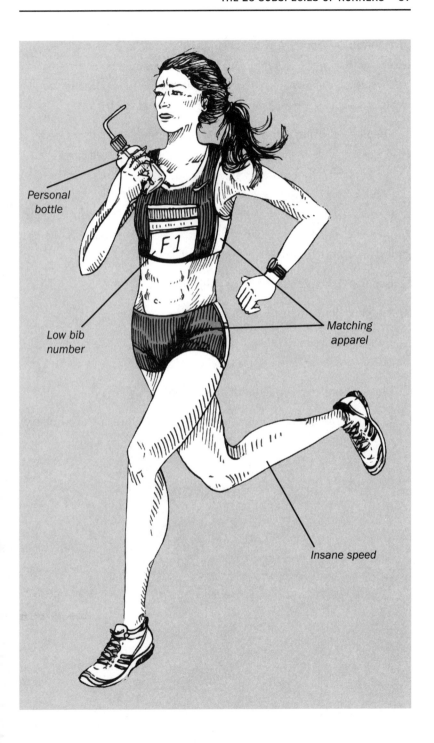

Personal
bottle

Low bib
number

Matching
apparel

Insane speed

☐ **Habitat:** The front of any race; behind microphones at news conferences; photo shoots. Geographically, North American Elites tend to cluster in Flagstaff, Arizona; Mammoth Lakes, California; Boulder, Colorado; and western Oregon. Some may migrate once a year or so to Africa.

☐ **Feeding behavior:** During a race, the Elite Runner will subsist on mystery liquids that he or she will suck from plastic bottles placed along the course. Researchers aren't sure what these liquids are, exactly, but based on the speed of those consuming them, they are assumed to count cocaine and pure corn syrup among their ingredients. Outside of competition, Elite Runners eat a variety of foods, just like anyone else. Their diets run the gamut from "very healthy" to "exceedingly healthy."

☐ **Sounds:** "Whoosh" (as they pass you)

☐ **Mating call:** "Want to share mystery liquids?"

☐ **Running style:** An Elite Runner in motion, at any speed, is pure elegance. Zero wasted effort. It's like they're floating.

☐ **Closest relatives:** The Serious Runner; the Grizzled Vet

☐ **Enemies and threats:** Time's slow, steady march; career-ending injury

WARNING!

While watching an Elite Runner run will amaze and inspire you, it may also leave you feeling like your own running form is crap. Which, let's face it, it is.

The High-Intensity Cross-Trainer

Lopus explosivus

At first blush, the High-Intensity Cross-Trainer has something in common with the Bucket Lister—namely, they both see running as a means to an end. But whereas the Bucket Lister uses running to achieve a life goal—i.e., doing a marathon—the High-Intensity Cross-Trainer uses it to INCINERATE CALORIES in the MOST EFFICIENT MANNER POSSIBLE, the better to PUSH THE BODY TO ITS ABSOLUTE LIMITS.[6]

It is believed that the High-Intensity Cross-Trainer is a mutated, amped-up version of the Fitness Runner—in the vernacular, "a Fitness Runner on steroids." In no way is this meant to impugn the character of the High-Intensity Cross-Trainer or to suggest that he is juiced to the gills.[7]

☐ **Distinguishing characteristics:** Fingerless gloves; compression sleeves; scary-looking "training mask" that is said to simulate high-altitude conditions

☐ **Appearance:** Jacked; hungry; visible veins

☐ **Habitat:** CrossFit gyms;[8] supplement stores; any place there are stairs or large truck tires

---

6 The High-Intensity Cross-Trainer is an ALL CAPS sort of runner.
7 And this is not to suggest that High-Intensity Cross-Trainers have actual gills. They do not. Yet.
8 I refuse to call them "boxes."

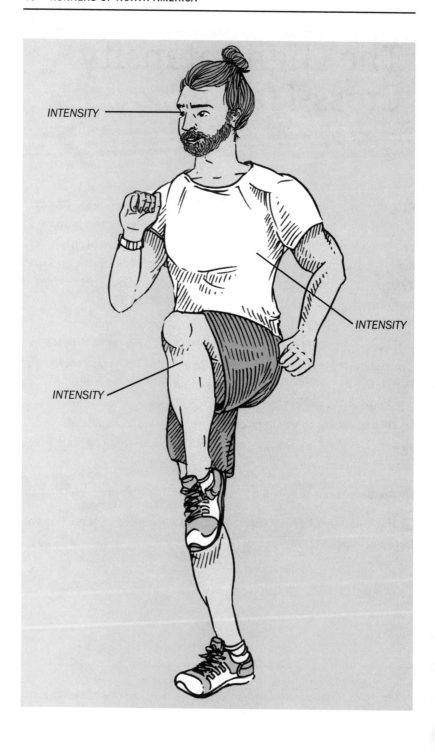

☐ **Feeding behavior:** Some High-Intensity Cross-Trainers are very particular about what they eat, favoring carefully blended smoothies and broiled, skinless chicken breasts. Others have diets that revolve around verbs like "scarf," "wolf," "chug," and "destroy." E.g.,

> High-Intensity Cross-Trainer #1: "Dudes, I just DESTROYED a plate of spicy wings."

> High-Intensity Cross-Trainer #2: "Bro! Here, CHUG this Mountain Dew!"

> High-Intensity Cross-Trainer #3: "CHUG! CHUG! CHUG!"

☐ **Sounds:** Heavy breathing; slap of high fives; chugging; scarfing

☐ **Mating call:** "GRRRRAAAAAAH!"

☐ **Running style:** INTENSE bursts of INTENSITY, often punctuated by "GRRRRAAAAAAH!"

☐ **Closest relatives:** The Fitness Runner

☐ **Enemies and threats:** Bogus supplements; catastrophic muscle or tendon injuries; long-distance runs

WARNING!

An especially "stoked" High-Intensity Cross-Trainer may attempt to bench-press or caber-toss you or your companions without provocation. If this happens, go limp and pretend to sleep. Eventually the High-Intensity Cross-Trainer will lose interest and move on.

The Adventure Racer

Lopus adrenalinus

If the Adventure Racer were a car, he would be a Jeep Wrangler that deliberately has not been washed in months. If he were a condiment, he would be Sriracha hot sauce. If he were a body of water, he would be Class IV rapids.

The point is this: The Adventure Racer craves adventure. He seeks novelty and thrills, to the extent that he will actually pay for the privilege of slogging through icy water and possibly being electrocuted. He is also a very social creature, which is what distinguishes the Adventure Racer from other sports-related species such as, say, the Free Solo Rock Climber.

If it weren't for adventure runs—"mud and obstacle" events, e.g., the Tough Mudder and Spartan Race series—it is likely that the Adventure Racer would run very little, if at all. For this reason, certain other runner subspecies look askance at the Adventure Racer. But the fact remains, the Adventure Racer does indeed run. (Often a runner may begin his or her life as an Adventure Racer before morphing into a different subspecies altogether.) Hence his inclusion in this guidebook.

☐ **Distinguishing characteristics:** Zest for life; Jeep Wrangler that deliberately has not been washed in months

☐ **Appearance:** The Adventure Racer opts for snug running attire, as it performs best in wet, muddy conditions (and under low-strung barbed wire); even if the weather is quite hot, he may wear grippy gloves while competing, to protect his hands and to make slick obstacles and ropes easier to handle.

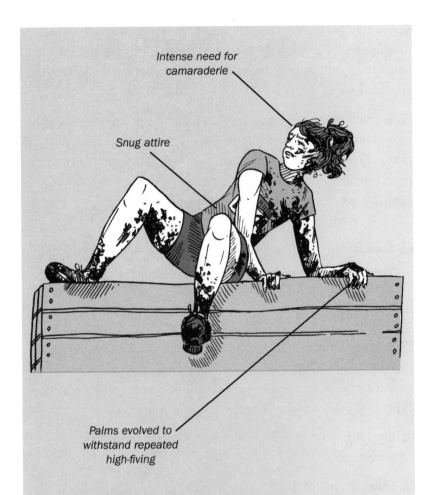

Intense need for camaraderie

Snug attire

Palms evolved to withstand repeated high-fiving

WARNING!

Because his need for intensity extends even to greetings, the Adventure Racer may unwittingly crush the smaller bones of your hand while shaking it. Under no circumstances should you permit an Adventure Racer to give you a bear hug. Helpful suggestions that the Adventure Racer's Jeep Wrangler could use a wash may be met with anger.

☐ **Habitat:** The gym; outdoors, flipping over enormous tractor tires or running up and down steps; cubicle or other nondescript office environment, where he or she toils away 8 or so hours each weekday, wishing he or she were somewhere else. Anywhere else.

☐ **Feeding behavior:** Because the Adventure Racer is drawn to intensity, he is a fan of hot sauce, and the hotter the better. Beyond that, his diet mimics that of other subspecies that favor short, intense running over longer, slower, steady-state running—this means a focus not on food but on Nutrition, with a weakness for powdered supplements and things like whey. Also beer.

☐ **Sounds:** During training and racing, the Adventure Racer communicates largely through a series of grunts and other guttural sounds; other times, he sounds perfectly normal.

☐ **Mating call:** "Wanna get dirty?"

☐ **Running style:** The Adventure Racer in motion may closely resemble the High-Intensity Cross-Trainer—or, to a lesser degree, the Fitness Runner—insofar as they rely on relatively short bursts of intense speed and/or power to get them where they need to go.

☐ **Closest relatives:** The High-Intensity Cross-Trainer; the Fitness Runner; the Bucket Lister

☐ **Enemies and threats:** Fly-by-night adventure race companies that collect entry fees then cancel the race; sudden, catastrophic injury; electrocution

The Dramatic Weight Loss Runner

Lopus saladus

The Dramatic Weight Loss Runner appears happy and fit, but this is not his defining trait. His defining trait is that before he started running, the Dramatic Weight Loss Runner did not appear fit or even all that happy, even if he is smiling in photos. Thanks to running, the Dramatic Weight Loss Runner has lost a ton of weight[9] and has never felt better. Because of this, he radiates gratitude and beneficence.

More than any other subspecies, the Dramatic Weight Loss Runner serves as an inspiration—not only to other runners but also to normal humans. "If the Dramatic Weight Loss Runner can do it, so can you." That is the uplifting message of the Dramatic Weight Loss Runner.

☐ **Distinguishing characteristics:** Before-and-after photos; genuine sense of satisfaction; aura of persistent determination

☐ **Appearance:** Clear eyes; loose clothing

☐ **Habitat:** Supermarket produce section; local running store, where he is picking up his bib number for that weekend's 5-K and perusing any new stability shoes on display

☐ **Feeding behavior:** The Dramatic Weight Loss Runner is very particular about what he or she eats, and understandably so; for this subspecies, his or her former, large self always seems just a carton of ice cream away. For this reason, the Dramatic Weight Loss Runner favors a diet rich in vegetables, low-fat dairy products, fish, and skinless chicken breasts. Also, the Dramatic Weight Loss Runner is never far from an enormous water bottle.

9 *And has the old pants to prove it.*

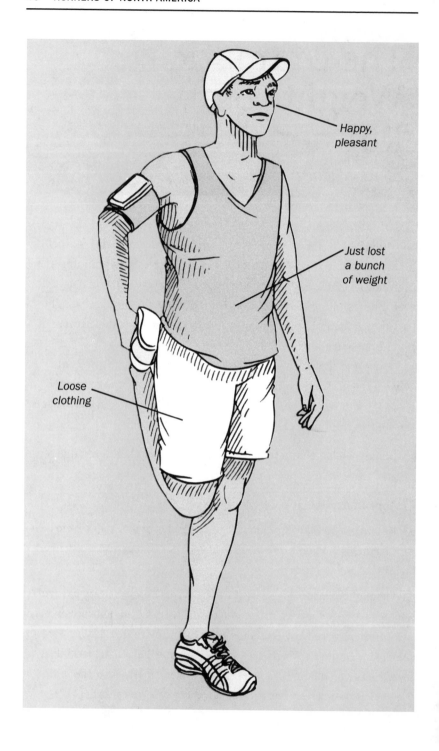

Happy, pleasant

Just lost a bunch of weight

Loose clothing

Sounds: "Could I get the dressing on the side?" ... "I've never felt better!" ... "No, it's me—Dominick![10] Yeah, I just lost a bunch of weight!"

Mating call: "Wanna see my 'fat pants'?"

Running style: Slow but determined; cheerful, too—the Dramatic Weight Loss Runner is just happy to be running at all.[11]

Closest relatives: The Club Runner; the Mom Runner; the Dad Runner

Enemies and threats: The Serious Runner; the Trail Runner; free breakfast buffets

WARNING!

Merely being in the presence of a Dramatic Weight Loss Runner may obliterate your own excuses—"I can't run" ... "Running is bad for your knees" ... etc.—in an instant, leaving you with no valid reasons not to put on your running shoes and head out the door.

---

10 Most, but not all, Dramatic Weight Loss Runners are named Dominick.
11 In this way, Dramatic Weight Loss Runners have a lesson for all of us.

The Barefoot Runner

Lopus naturalis

Long ago, all runners were, by default, Barefoot Runners. Then humans invented shoes and began wearing them everywhere. Runners, who have a gift for mimicry, soon followed suit, and Barefoot Runners became virtually extinct.

Not entirely extinct, though—a handful of Barefoot Runners survived. They must have mated furiously, because early in the 21st century their numbers exploded.[12] This population growth coincided with the publication of Chris McDougall's 2009 book *Born to Run,* which describes the Tarahumara Indian tribe in the Mexican Copper Canyons, whose members routinely run long distances without shoes or even fanny packs.

Most Barefoot Runners are quiet and pleasant, but some are quite vocal and easily angered when they feel they're being threatened. Especially on the Internet.

☐ **Distinguishing characteristics:** A conspicuous lack of shoes; zealotry; unmistakable—and vaguely menacing—"slap, slap" sound as they approach you from behind while running on pavement

☐ **Appearance:** Almost always male; lean and tan; calloused (and surprisingly clean) feet; absence of sock tan lines

☐ **Habitat:** Smooth, paved paths; groomed trails; Chris McDougall speaking engagements

---

12 Scholars estimate that as many as 250 Barefoot Runners exist today!

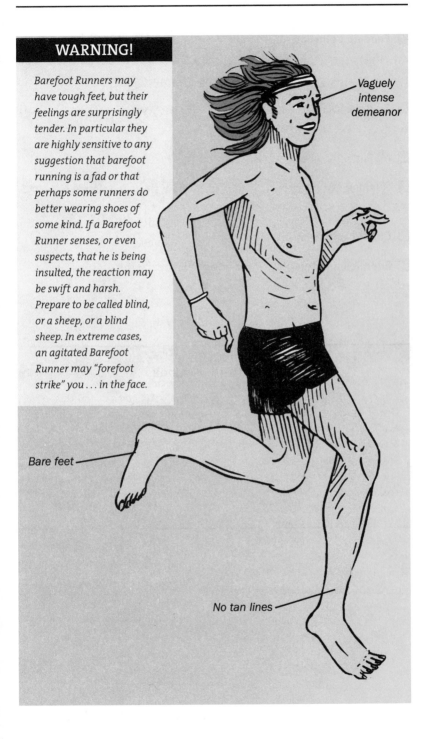

WARNING!

Barefoot Runners may have tough feet, but their feelings are surprisingly tender. In particular they are highly sensitive to any suggestion that barefoot running is a fad or that perhaps some runners do better wearing shoes of some kind. If a Barefoot Runner senses, or even suspects, that he is being insulted, the reaction may be swift and harsh. Prepare to be called blind, or a sheep, or a blind sheep. In extreme cases, an agitated Barefoot Runner may "forefoot strike" you . . . in the face.

Vaguely intense demeanor

Bare feet

No tan lines

☐ **Feeding behavior:** Many, though certainly not all, Barefoot Runners are either vegetarians or followers of a Paleo-style diet. Scientists speculate that this may contribute to their often-gruff demeanor.

☐ **Sounds:** "Good luck with those FOOT COFFINS you're wearing!" ... "I haven't been injured in years!"

☐ **Mating call:** "Nice sandals."

☐ **Running style:** Barefoot, usually with short, shuffling steps—THE WAY NATURE INTENDED

☐ **Closest relatives:** The Trail Runner

☐ **Enemies and threats:** Broken glass; sharp rocks; the running shoe industry, aka "Big Shoe"

"Barefoot Shoes": A Running Paradox

One of the strangest developments in modern Barefoot Running is the introduction of "barefoot running shoes." These paradoxically named products are meant to offer some measure of protection for the Barefoot Runner while delivering a barefoot "feel" while running. Among the most popular of these are Vibram FiveFingers—thin, glovelike footwear with individual compartments for each toe. Scientists theorize that these shoes have the added benefit of discouraging inter-species breeding, as no one except a fellow Barefoot Runner would mate with someone wearing them.

The Mom Runner

Lopus matercula

Don't let the name fool you. The Mom Runner is not merely a runner who happens to be a mother; she is a very specific kind of runner who happens to be a mother.

Mom Runners come from all walks of life, though—as with most runners—they tend to be middle- to upper-middle class and in reasonably good shape even before they take up running. Some Mom Runners started their running lives as Fitness Runners or Fashion Mag Runners; others simply woke up one day and found themselves in the body of a Mom Runner. What they all have in common is a love of running. And of wine.

Mom Runners tend to move in packs.

☐ **Distinguishing characteristics:** T-shirt or hoodie declaring herself a "badass"; ponytail (while running); jogging stroller; minivan with an I RUN LIKE A GIRL sticker; habit of mentioning how she got her run in SO EARLY, before the kids woke up, making you feel like a slug

☐ **Appearance:** The Mom Runner comes in many shapes and sizes and generally appears happy, especially while she's running; in general she looks great, though she will insist that she looks great "for her age."

☐ **Habitat:** Comfortable suburban home decorated tastefully, including conspicuous signs of the Mom Runner—e.g., handmade race medal rack, race T-shirt quilt, yoga mat, wine fridge; preschools, kindergartens, and elementary schools, where they may be seen lingering after drop-off, wearing tights and holding Starbucks cups

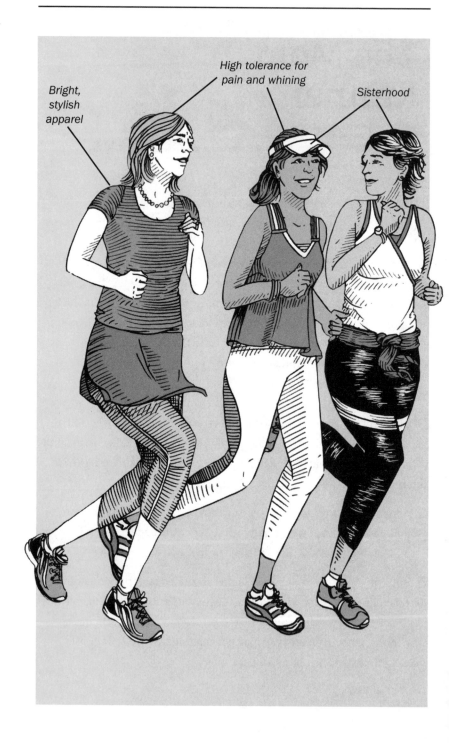

☐ **Feeding behavior:** The Mom Runner enjoys wine. Beyond that, she eats fairly healthfully, because she tries to feed her children healthfully and she wants to set a good example. But she is not above devouring a cupcake over the kitchen sink when no one is looking.

☐ **Sounds:** "Should we open another bottle?"

☐ **Mating call:** N/A. This is someone's *mother* we're talking about.

☐ **Running style:** Light and smooth; happy. Because she is educated and conscientious, the Mom Runner has done her homework and generally knows what she's doing.

☐ **Closest relatives:** The Club Runner; the Fashion Mag Runner

☐ **Enemies and threats:** Restaurant brunches that offer unlimited mimosas

---

WARNING!

May call you "girlfriend," even if you are not in fact her girlfriend.

The Dad Runner

Lopus paternus

As with the Mom Runner, the Dad Runner is not just any runner who happens to be a father but a specific *kind* of runner who happens to be a father.

Dad Runners may run with others, including other Dad Runners, but are equally content to run alone. (Or to run with their offspring, in a jogging stroller.) In this way they differ from Mom Runners, for whom running is a crucial social outlet.

Many Dad Runners are stubbornly competitive—a vestige of their days as a Fitness Runner or Serious Runner.

☐ **Distinguishing characteristics:** Reluctance to let you pass them; jogging stroller; years-old race shirt (he hasn't had as much time for racing since the kids came along); sensible car with running stickers (Mom has the van)

☐ **Appearance:** Small but unmistakable gut[13]

☐ **Habitat:** Comfortable suburban home decorated tastefully; garage or basement of same home

☐ **Feeding behavior:** The Dad Runner is a scavenger, eating whatever he can find, wherever he can find it—from sushi to nachos, from his kids' untouched peanut butter toast to Lunchable remnants. Also he enjoys beer.

☐ **Sounds:** Loud belching

☐ **Mating call:** N/A. He's married.

---

13 *He knows. He's working on it.*

☐ **Running style:** Upright; slightly tense; brisk—just a little bit faster than he should be going

☐ **Closest relatives:** The Mom Runner; the Serious Runner

☐ **Enemies and threats:** Shin splints; spit-up (from his child)

WARNING!

Running alongside the Dad Runner, you might find yourself drawn into an involuntary race. The Dad Runner used to be fast, dammit.

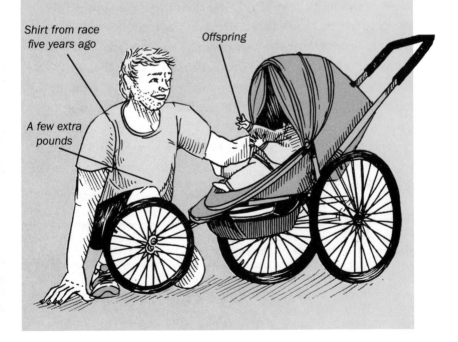

Shirt from race five years ago

Offspring

A few extra pounds

The Grizzled Vet

Lopus veteranus

Encountering a Grizzled Vet is as close as you can come to traveling back in time and speaking with a runner from an earlier era, without employing an actual time machine.[14] These fascinating creatures are, as the name implies, old. They also tend to be deeply tanned, or to show the effects of decades spent deeply tanned. This means they are also creased in very interesting ways.

At the same time, the Grizzled Vet is strong and energetic. Often he or she can run you into the ground and celebrate afterward with a few one-handed pushups. The Grizzled Vet takes great delight in this.

You can punch a Grizzled Vet in the stomach with no apparent ill effects. In fact, the Grizzled Vet might insist you do so. "Give me your best shot," the Grizzled Vet will say, slapping his own gut. "Go on. Do it."[15]

Whether you punch him or not, the Grizzled Vet may also say, "(Blank) years old, still hard as a rock." The reason he will say "blank" is that he has forgotten his age. While the Grizzled Vet's abdomen is in fine shape, his mind may not be.

Still, the Grizzled Vet's love for running is as strong as ever. For this reason, he is a source of great inspiration for other runners, who often refer to him as "the real deal."

---

14 If you did have an actual time machine, of course, you could also travel forward in time, which would be a lot more interesting. Topic for discussion: How might runners look hundreds of years from now? Will their running shoes be super-fancy? Will they have "26.2" stickers on their nuclear-powered hover cars? Will they be hairless?

15 Do not punch a Grizzled Vet—in the stomach or elsewhere—uninvited. That is called battery and can land you in court.

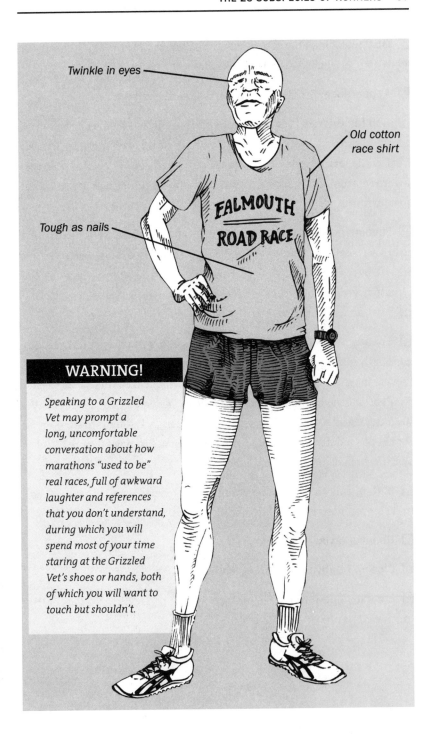

Twinkle in eyes

Old cotton race shirt

Tough as nails

FALMOUTH ROAD RACE

WARNING!

Speaking to a Grizzled Vet may prompt a long, uncomfortable conversation about how marathons "used to be" real races, full of awkward laughter and references that you don't understand, during which you will spend most of your time staring at the Grizzled Vet's shoes or hands, both of which you will want to touch but shouldn't.

☐ **Distinguishing characteristics:** Doesn't have time for your bullshit Walkman or whatever that doohickey is.

☐ **Appearance:** Grizzled; old; cotton race shirts; mischievous eyes

☐ **Habitat:** Grizzled Vets love to race, so you will find them at just about any local running event. For an up-close look, linger after the race. Grizzled Vets, while relatively small in number, are heavily represented at postrace awards presentations, where they are sometimes guaranteed an award just by finishing.

☐ **Feeding behavior:** The Grizzled Vet eats just like he always has, which is to say he eats what he wants, when he wants, goddammit. Before a race, he will have a cup of coffee (black) and a Centrum Silver multivitamin. The Grizzled Vet is the only subspecies of runner who refers to candy, pastries, desserts, and so on as "sweets."

☐ **Sounds:** Some Grizzled Vets make strange sounds while running hard, especially during a race. These sounds can range from "deep wheeze" to "severe moan" to "rhythmic grunt." Or some unique combination of these. Don't be alarmed. It may sound as if they are in distress, but usually they aren't. Scientists theorize that Grizzled Vets use such sounds to frighten would-be predators, or to announce their presence to other Grizzled Vets within earshot.

☐ **Mating call:** N/A. Almost invariably, the Grizzled Vet is either married or no longer interested in sex. Or both.

☐ **Running style:** Aggressive

☐ **Closest relatives:** The Serious Runner

☐ **Enemies and threats:** Technology; themed runs ("Mud," "Color," etc.); anyone who runs a race with a phone

The 7:00-Minute-Mile Guy

Lopus mono velocitus

For all outward appearances, the 7:00-Minute-Mile Guy—they are almost always male—is strikingly similar to the Serious Runner. They both run a lot and are "serious" about it. They both tend to be young, relatively speaking. Both are fast. But they differ in two crucial and related ways:

1. While the Serious Runner employs things like speed training and rest days, the 7:00-Minute-Mile Guy does not.

2. The Serious Runner tapers before a race, arrives at the starting line fresh and rested, and has a mile-by-mile strategy to reach his goal. The 7:00-Minute-Mile Guy, on the other hand, barely tapers at all and arrives at the starting line still "feeling it" from the previous weekend's 20-miler. His mile-by-mile plan is as follows: Run at a 7:00-minute pace. To his credit, the 7:00-Minute-Mile Guy will follow this plan to a T. Until he can't.

This is the defining trait of the 7:00-Minute-Mile Guy—he runs the exact same pace (usually around 7:00 per mile), no matter what. If 7:00-Minute-Mile Guy were a manual-transmission car, he would be in third gear all the time, whether in a fast-food drive-through or on the interstate.

☐ **Distinguishing characteristics:** Never warms up. Runs 7:00-minute-per-mile pace at all times, regardless of distance, purpose of run, or company. Wonders why his latest marathon ended in disappointment, when he was right on 7:00-minute pace until "the wheels came off."

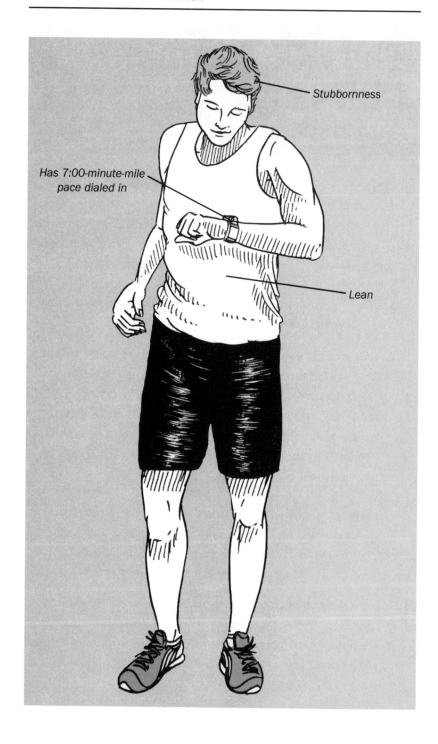

☐ **Appearance:** Lean; steely expression

☐ **Habitat:** Seen often on treadmills at the gym or on multiuse paths

☐ **Feeding behavior:** Varies widely. 7:00-Minute-Mile Guys may be very particular about what they eat and when they eat it ("If I'm going to run a 7:00-minute pace, I need to eat well"), but they are just as likely to pay little to no attention to diet ("I run a 7:00-minute pace; I can eat whatever I want"). The 7:00-Minute-Mile Guy is very inconsistent. Except when it comes to pace.

☐ **Sounds:** "Hey, we averaged a 7:00-minute pace. Cool."

☐ **Mating call:** "I'm pretty fast."

☐ **Running style:** Pretty fast, all the time

☐ **Closest relatives:** The Serious Runner

☐ **Enemies and threats:** Age; burnout; 400-meter repeats

WARNING!

Runs with the 7:00-Minute-Mile Guy will be annoying at best and unsustainable at worst—unless you are also a 7:00-Minute-Mile Guy.

The Gear Addict

Lopus productus

The Gear Addict, as the name implies, loves gear. He cannot get enough. If you were to enter the home of a Gear Addict and open a hall closet, you would run a real risk of being buried, cartoon-style, in an avalanche of stuff falling out—watches, foam rollers, hydration packs, hats, LED-studded hats, activity-tracking bracelets, wireless headphones, ice packs, windproof vests, featherweight jackets, water bottles, headlamps, tights, shorts, yoga mats, waist packs, armband iPhone cases, compression socks, $200 sunglasses,[16] and an incredible number of running shoes, many of which are still in their boxes.

In a cartoon, of course, a bowling ball would then slowly roll off a shelf and onto your head. Luckily, few Gear Addict runners today are also into bowling.

At least 45 percent of the Gear Addict's disposable income goes toward the purchase of running gear. He knows this because he has an app that tracks his spending, and he regularly pores over that data, along with his mileage (daily, weekly, monthly, year-to-date), pace, elevation gains and losses, weight, body fat percentage, and the miles logged in each of his 23 pairs of shoes. For this reason, he is on a first-name basis with the staff of his local REI store and the managers and assistant managers of every specialty running store in his zip code.

On a related note, the Gear Addict can be a useful source of slightly used running gear, as he tends to discard stuff the moment a newer model comes along.

---

16 He will insist on calling them "eyewear."

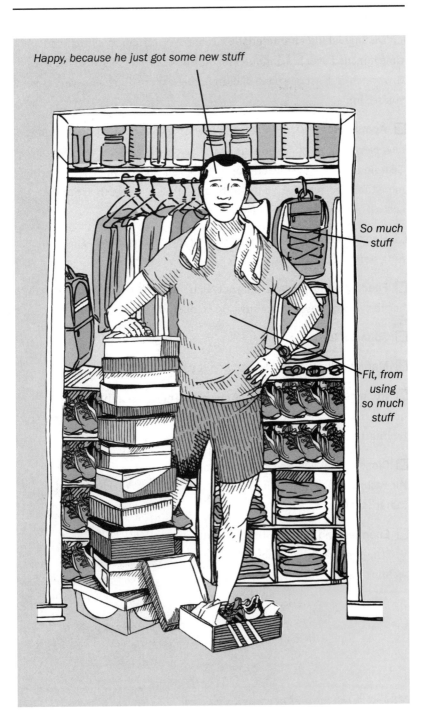

☐ **Distinguishing characteristics:** Poor posture, from spending so much time hunched over his computer reading 6,000-word reviews of the latest GPS watch; at least one piece of brand-new gear on his person every time you see him

☐ **Appearance:** Smiling, because every time you see him he has a brand-new piece of gear; fit, because he actually does *use* all that new gear. The Gear Addict is pretty much the only runner subspecies you'll see wearing more than one watch at a time, as he often likes to gauge their accuracy against one another in a road test.

☐ **Habitat:** Running gear Web sites; running gear retail Web sites; running stores

☐ **Feeding behavior:** While it's not "gear," per se, the Gear Addict usually has the very newest sports nutrition products on or near him.

☐ **Sounds:** "Is that new?"

☐ **Mating call:** "Wow, I'd love to unbox *you*."

☐ **Running style:** Varies, but the one constant is that it involves frequently checking in with his various pieces of gear—adjusting, calibrating, fooling around with, or simply admiring

☐ **Closest relatives:** The Fitness Runner; the Fashion Mag Runner; the Serial Marathoner

☐ **Enemies and threats:** The Grizzled Vet; the Barefoot Runner; obsolete technology

WARNING!

When he is standing very still, the Gear Addict may be mistaken for a mannequin displaying the season's newest running accessories. Keep this in mind the next time you're tempted to fondle a mannequin.[17]

---

17 *I'm not the only one who fondles mannequins . . . right?*

The Charity Runner

Lopus altruistus

The Charity Runner runs for something bigger than herself. Sure, she enjoys running's many benefits—health, happiness, camaraderie, and so on. But what drives her is the "high" she gets not only from running but also from running to help others.

Certain other subspecies[18] treat the Charity Runner with suspicion or even contempt. No one is sure why. But it's a real bummer.

☐ **Distinguishing characteristics:** Cheerful; hopeful; has "got this"

☐ **Appearance:** Big smile; temporary tattoo; running shirt with charity's logo

☐ **Habitat:** Long runs with fellow Charity Runners; posing for group photos; social media

☐ **Feeding behavior:** The Charity Runner's diet consists chiefly of the pretzels, gummy worms, and Twizzlers provided during group runs.

☐ **Sounds:** "Woooo!"

☐ **Mating call:** "I give till it hurts."

☐ **Running style:** Dogged; joyful; selfless

18 *We're looking at you, Serious Runner.*

☐ **Closest relatives:** The Club Runner; the Bucket Lister

☐ **Enemies and threats:** The Serious Runner; stingy relatives

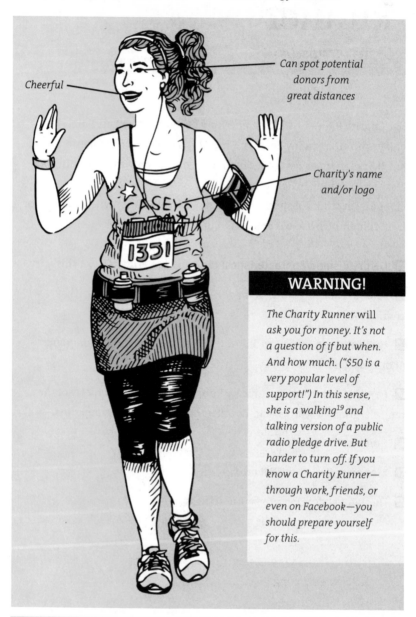

Cheerful

Can spot potential donors from great distances

Charity's name and/or logo

WARNING!

The Charity Runner will ask you for money. It's not a question of if but when. And how much. ("$50 is a very popular level of support!") In this sense, she is a walking[19] and talking version of a public radio pledge drive. But harder to turn off. If you know a Charity Runner— through work, friends, or even on Facebook—you should prepare yourself for this.

---

19 Well, running.

The Serial Marathoner

Lopus pheidippidus

Serial Marathoners are the chain smokers of the running world. They've registered for their next race—maybe for their next several races—even before they've finished the one they're currently working on.[20]

But running isn't smoking. Running is healthy! And so the Serial Marathoner forges ahead, until death or debilitating injury stops her.

More than just about any other subspecies, the Serial Marathoner uses running to define herself. Other runners may run marathons. But the Serial Marathoner *is a marathoner.*

If you need advice on running marathons, it probably goes without saying, you're going to want to ask a Serial Marathoner. Just do so carefully. (See "Warning!" on page 68.)

Because they travel so frequently, Serial Marathoners also happen to be very knowledgeable about airports, current TSA policies, hotel deals, carry-on-compliant luggage, and those little U-shaped pillows that wrap around your neck.

☐ **Distinguishing characteristics:** Crazy eyes; a compulsion to affix "26.2" stickers to every available surface (she may buy them by the gross); awful toenails, even for a runner; travel-size foam roller

☐ **Appearance:** Lean; intense; wearing running shoes that are either extremely worn (for obvious reasons) or extremely new (because she just retired a pair that was extremely worn). Because the Serial Marathoner's race-shirt collection has grown like ivy in her closet, choking off other, weaker forms of clothing, she wears race shirts almost exclusively.

---

20 *In extreme cases, a Serial Marathoner may be registered for 10 or more future marathons, making her less like a chain smoker and more like those guys you see in* Guinness World Records *with their mouths crammed with 110 cigarettes.*

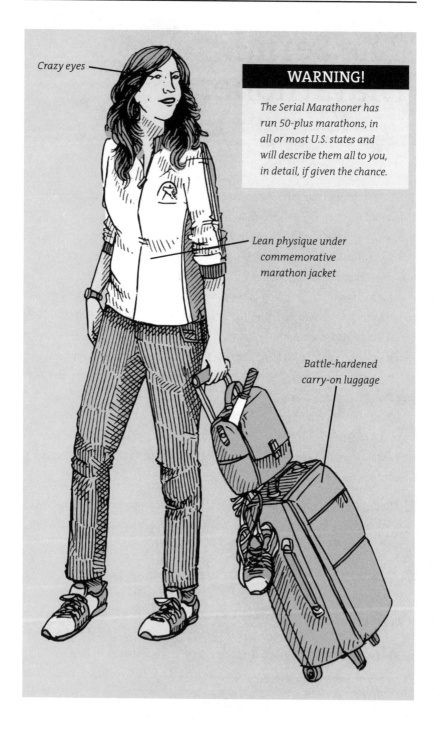

Crazy eyes

WARNING!

The Serial Marathoner has run 50-plus marathons, in all or most U.S. states and will describe them all to you, in detail, if given the chance.

Lean physique under commemorative marathon jacket

Battle-hardened carry-on luggage

☐ **Habitat:** Online forums devoted to running marathons in general or certain marathons in particular; marathon expos; marathon starting corrals; marathon finish areas; ice baths

☐ **Feeding behavior:** Much of the Serial Marathoner's diet consists of foods eaten just before a marathon, during the marathon, or after the marathon. Roughly 15 percent of her total calories may come exclusively from celebratory cheeseburgers and beer consumed after a marathon. The Serial Marathoner is also a "grazer," however—she can often be seen snacking on tiny bags of pretzels, apples, bananas, bagels, granola bars, and cartons of coconut water, all of which she has stockpiled from numerous trips through marathon finisher chutes.

☐ **Sounds:** "Hey, I've run that marathon."

☐ **Mating call:** "After my next marathon, honey, I promise."

☐ **Running style:** Usually very fluid and economical. Not always, though. Certain Serial Marathoners appear to get through so many 26.2-mile races not because of their running form but in spite of it.

☐ **Closest relatives:** The Serious Runner; the Club Runner

☐ **Enemies and threats:** Prohibitively high airfares; flight delays; serious injury; neglected spouses who are one "long run" away from piling all of the Serial Marathoner's running shoes up, dousing them with kerosene, and lighting a match

The Trail Runner

Lopus granolus

These shy, slender creatures, while relatively small in number, are among running's most graceful and exotic specimens. Because of their quick reflexes, speed over tricky terrain, and instinctive distrust of humans, Trail Runners are difficult to spot and even more difficult to photograph. Sightings in the wild are rare but can be very rewarding. (For tips on sighting and photographing Trail Runners, see page 134.)

As their name suggests, Trail Runners are found exclusively or nearly exclusively on trails and paths, and in other "nature"-based locations.[21] In rare cases, you may encounter a Trail Runner in a suburban setting, looking frightened and confused. If that happens, experts recommend avoiding eye contact and contacting your local wildlife agency.

A Trail Runner found in an urban environment may have to be sedated and airlifted to safety.

☐ **Distinguishing characteristics:** Facial hair (males); 2.5 percent body fat; eyes that seem to see right through you; water bottle strapped to hand

☐ **Appearance:** Tall, thin, lean, tan; often shirtless; filthy ankles and shins. Trail Runners are roughly 75 percent more likely than other runners to have one or more tattoos.

☐ **Habitat:** *Nature*, man. Nothing like it.

---

21 *Logging roads present a challenge to the Trail Runner. On one hand, they're roads, and roads are not natural or beautiful or serene. On the other, they're found in natural settings, such as large forests. On the third hand, they were created for the purposes of logging, which is antithetical to everything the Trail Runner stands for. On the fourth hand, perhaps the Trail Runner's appropriation of these roads itself is a powerful statement to the logging and timber industry that he will not be cowed by Big Lumber. These are the sorts of things a Trail Runner can ponder during a 2-hour run alone in the woods.*

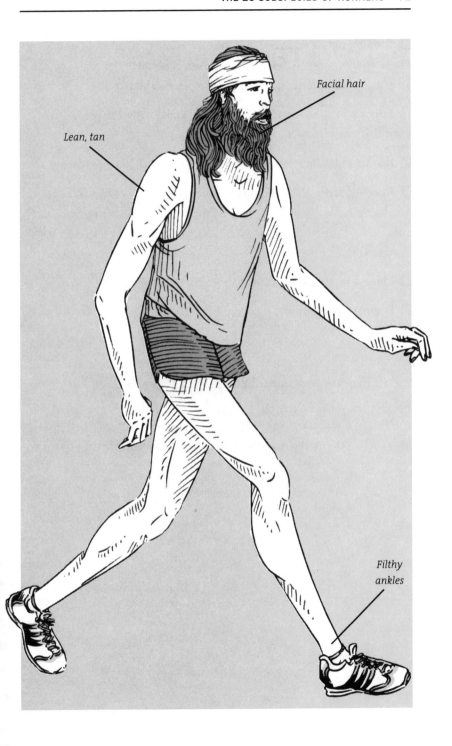

☐ **Feeding behavior:** In line with their devotion to nature and simplicity, Trail Runners gravitate toward simple diets of berries, nuts, and vegetables. They may occasionally trap and eat a fish or small bird.

☐ **Sounds:** Just the sounds of his footfalls and the rhythm of his own breathing; the phrase "right on"

☐ **Mating call:** More rhythmic breathing, but faster and more urgent

☐ **Running style:** A Trail Runner in full flight is the very picture of grace. Because he has evolved to navigate terrain filled with rocks, roots, holes, streams, and various forms of wildlife, and to do so nearly unconsciously, he runs with an ease and fluidity that is the envy of all other runners.

☐ **Closest relatives:** The Ultra Runner; the Grizzled Vet

☐ **Enemies and threats:** Roots; snakes; ticks; asphalt; mountain bikers

WARNING!

Some Trail Runners are capable of near-lethal levels of contempt if they feel you aren't respecting Trail Culture. Non–Trail Runners who blunder into Trail Runners' territory wearing, say, a Color Run tee and jogging three abreast may be mauled and buried hastily under a pile of large rocks. Or badly injured and left to return to civilization, as a warning to others.

The Ultra Runner

Lopus extremus

Merriam-Webster defines *ultra* as "going beyond others or beyond due limit." While this certainly applies to the Ultra Runner—in the simplest terms, an Ultra Runner is one who runs ultra distances—it falls far short of painting a full picture of this "ultra"-rare subspecies.

An "ultra distance," technically speaking, is anything beyond a marathon—i.e., anything longer than 26.2 miles. Ultra Runners typically run distances that aren't just longer than that but much longer; events of 100-K (62 miles), 100 miles, or more aren't uncommon for the Ultra Runner. (These events are often, though not always, held on trails, leading casual observers to mistakenly identify Ultra Runners as Trail Runners.)

Running that long or that far seems insane, not only to humans but also to other runners. It isn't, though. At least not literally—brain autopsies of Ultra Runners[22] suggest that insanity is no more prevalent in this subspecies than in any other.

So what exactly *does* motivate the Ultra Runner, if not a diseased brain? Scientists aren't sure. And the runners themselves aren't likely to volunteer an answer—as a subspecies, Ultra Runners tend to be quiet, reserved, and humble to a fault. (Particularly when contrasted with, for instance, the Adventure Racer or the Serious Runner.)

It's possible we may never know what makes them run. This only adds to the allure of these enigmatic creatures.

---

22 *These procedures were halted in the mid-1970s, when critics pointed out that they were decimating an already small population of Ultra Runners.*

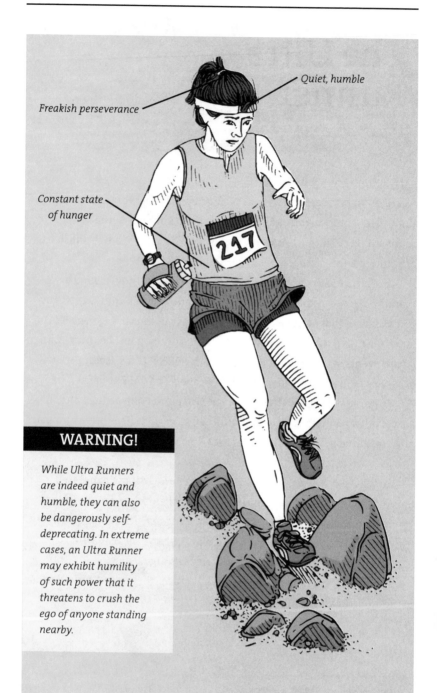

Quiet, humble

Freakish perseverance

Constant state
of hunger

217

WARNING!

*While Ultra Runners
are indeed quiet and
humble, they can also
be dangerously self-
deprecating. In extreme
cases, an Ultra Runner
may exhibit humility
of such power that it
threatens to crush the
ego of anyone standing
nearby.*

☐ **Distinguishing characteristics:** A near-total lack of free time; constant hunger; large belt buckles

☐ **Appearance:** Other than a sleek, slender body, the Ultra Runner appears remarkably . . . normal. Meeting one in passing, you would never know that he or she routinely runs 30 or 50 miles at a time, or more. Even other runners have a difficult time identifying Ultra Runners in their midst.

☐ **Habitat:** Roads, paths, trails, treadmills, airport concourses . . . anywhere they can squeeze some miles in; ultra events, either competing, volunteering, or "crewing" for a friend

☐ **Feeding behavior:** The Ultra Runner is famous for the amount of food she can put away. Especially while competing, she will resemble nothing so much as a roving eating machine, consuming just about anything in her path. Bystanders will marvel at how such a small runner can hold so much food.

☐ **Sounds:** Even with their sensitive recording equipment, scientists have yet to capture any sort of sound made by an Ultra Runner. That is how quiet and reserved they are.

☐ **Mating call:** N/A. Ultra Runners have neither the time nor the energy for this.

☐ **Running style:** In a word: *indefatigable*

☐ **Closest relatives:** The Trail Runner; the Grizzled Vet; the Irish novelist and playwright Samuel Beckett, whose line "I can't go on, I'll go on" would become a sort of unofficial motto and mantra for Ultra Runners everywhere

☐ **Enemies and threats:** Overuse injuries; hallucinations

The Kid Runner

Lopus juvenilis

Just as human children aren't simply miniature adults, the Kid Runner isn't simply a miniature runner. She is a subspecies unto herself. She may or may not grow up to become one of a number of other runner subspecies. In fact, she gives little to no thought to whether she'll be a runner in the future; all she knows is that she is running now and that she loves it.

This simple, innocent joy—and the accompanying presence of mind— is the essence of the Kid Runner.

It may go without saying, but other runners, and even many humans, find it impossible to watch Kid Runners out running and not feel inspired.

☐ **Distinguishing characteristics:** Unbridled joy

☐ **Appearance:** Big smile; baggy race T-shirt; footwear ranging from actual running shoes to sneakers to sandals

☐ **Habitat:** Kids races; playgrounds; parks; backyards

☐ **Feeding behavior:** Kid Runners eat just about anything a human kid might eat; because many of them are the children of runners, though, they may develop a taste for energy bars, bagels, and bananas.

☐ **Sounds:** Laughter

☐ **Mating call:** N/A

☐ **Running style:** Kid Runners don't care how they look while running, and it shows. While some may exhibit surprisingly good running form, many others are all over the place. They have fun anyway. Note that Kid

Runners, like many Newbie Runners, tend to have just two speeds when they run—sprint and plod. This makes a certain amount of sense, as Kid Runners are "newbies" by default.

☐ **Closest relatives:** Human children

☐ **Enemies and threats:** Video games; texting; the Internet; self-consciousness

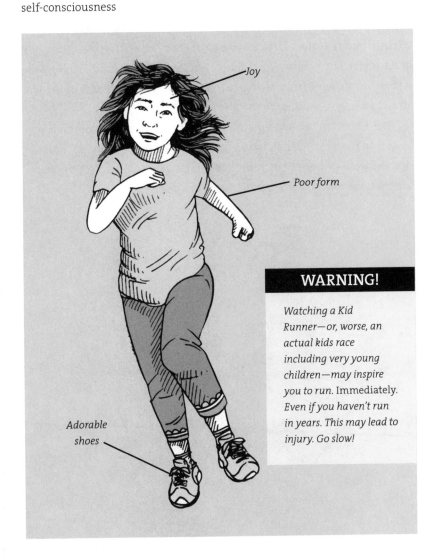

Joy

Poor form

Adorable shoes

WARNING!

Watching a Kid Runner—or, worse, an actual kids race including very young children—may inspire you to run. Immediately. Even if you haven't run in years. This may lead to injury. Go slow!

Zany Costumes: Not for Every Runner

The casual observer could be forgiven for assuming that the Costumed Runner is a subspecies unto itself. It is not.

While it is common to see costumes at any major race—and, increasingly, many smaller ones—the runners wearing them represent any number of subspecies. Why does a runner choose to race in a costume, when doing so is often hot, uncomfortable, and (in rare cases) even dangerous? Sometimes it is a stunt to raise money for charity. Sometimes it is the result of a drunken bet gone wrong. Some researchers speculate that the costume wearer has suffered (is suffering?) a mild psychotic episode or is trying to attract a mate, depending on the costume.

It is important to note that you will not see every subspecies among costumed runners. No matter how drunk or desperate for a mate, certain runners would sooner beat themselves unconscious with a Stick™ brand self-massage roller than wear a costume in a race.

Will You See This Runner in a Costume?

	YES	NO	MAYBE
THE NEWBIE		X	
THE "I'M NOT A REAL RUNNER" RUNNER			X
THE CLUB RUNNER			X
THE FITNESS RUNNER		X	
THE BUCKET LISTER			X
THE WEIRDO RUNNER	X		
THE FASHION MAG RUNNER		X	
THE SERIOUS RUNNER		X	
THE ELITE RUNNER		X	
THE HIGH-INTENSITY CROSS-TRAINER			X
THE ADVENTURE RACER			X
THE DRAMATIC WEIGHT LOSS RUNNER			X
THE BAREFOOT RUNNER		X	
THE MOM RUNNER			X
THE DAD RUNNER		X	
THE GRIZZLED VET		X	
THE 7:00-MINUTE-MILE GUY		X	
THE GEAR ADDICT		X	
THE CHARITY RUNNER	X		
THE SERIAL MARATHONER		X	
THE TRAIL RUNNER		X	
THE ULTRA RUNNER		X	
THE KID RUNNER	X		

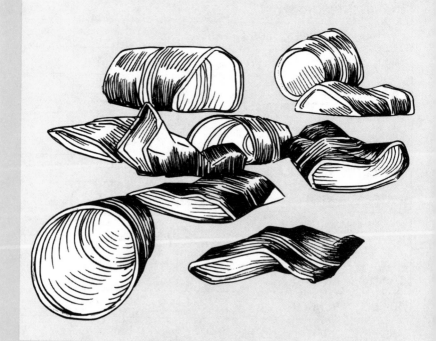

PART II

DID YOU KNOW?

As recently as the 1970s, runners could go 30 minutes or more without using sports drinks or energy gels to "refuel."

CHAPTER 3

DIET AND NUTRITION

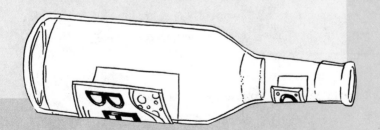

MANY RUNNERS HAVE A COMPLEX relationship with food, using it not just as sustenance but also as motivation and reward. In fact, just the thought of certain foods waiting for him at the finish can carry a runner for many miles. It is now believed that the first-ever "marathon" runner, the Greek hero Pheidippides, ran 26 miles to Athens not to share news of a military victory but because he was told there would be baklava.

Indeed, while some runners go by the motto "Live to Run, Run to Live," others maintain that they "Eat to Run and Run to Eat."

Dietary Habits: Three Major Types

Broadly speaking, runners may be divided into one of three dietary camps.

BIRDS

So named because they eat like birds. Not because they eat actual birds, or much of *any* sort of meat. These runners get plenty of protein through grains, legumes, and egg whites. What, you think they don't get enough protein? Well, they do, and they've *never felt better.* Birds are often vegetarians or vegans, or mostly so. In that case, of course, the egg whites are off the table. But they still get plenty of protein! Why do you care so much about protein? Stop obsessing over protein!

Here is what a typical meal might look like for a Bird:

O   Kale

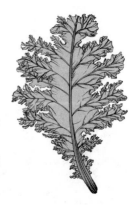

For a special treat, a Bird might "dress" her lunch with a teaspoon of olive oil or a squeeze of lemon juice. On the side.

A Bird not only avoids things like cookies but also makes a lot of noise about the fact that she avoids cookies. Typically this comes in the form of joking (not joking) panic ("Ack! Cookies! Get them away from me!") or self-flagellation

("Can't believe I ate a whole pancake! Must run 3 extra miles tonight!"), also in a joking (not joking) way.

The Bird loves a nice glass or three of red wine. Which is fine, because all she had for dinner was a big spoonful of hummus, and besides, red wine is good for you. Right?

PURITANS

For the Puritan, eating is less about enjoyment and more about calibrating the ingestion of micro- and macronutrients for optimal performance. Puritans often dispense with the word "food" altogether, instead calling the things they eat and drink "fuel." They think of their bodies as finely tuned machines. Would you put apple fritters into a finely tuned machine? Of course not. You put high-octane *fuel* into a finely tuned machine.

Except the true Puritan would not use the term "apple fritters." The true Puritan would use the word "crap" or "garbage" or, in extreme cases, "POISON," in all caps.

The Puritan loves to talk about fuel, especially with other Puritans. Topics of conversation might include:

O   This Banana: Too Large to Be Considered One Serving?

O   Instant Oatmeal: TOO MUCH SODIUM

O   How Many Grams of Carbs Should I Have the Morning of a Marathon?

O   What If This Large Banana Has Too Many Grams of Carbs? WHAT THEN?

O   Ways to Make Pizza More Joyless

The Puritan drinks mostly soy or almond milk, or filtered water. Puritans rarely smile.

NORMALS

When it comes to diet and nutrition, most runners are Normals. This means that they try to eat "right," whatever that might mean at any given

Q&A

Q: *I was runner-spotting in a local park recently when I noticed a specimen—I believe it was a Fitness Runner, though I can't be sure—slow down to remove a small, brightly colored object from a plastic wrapper. He then placed the object in his mouth and seemed to chew and swallow it. What was going on?*

—Mary, New York City

A: *What you saw was a runner eating mid-run. How exciting! Based on your description, it sounds like he was enjoying an "energy chew"—a curious blend of glucose syrup, gelatin, glycerin, carnauba wax, and artificial and natural flavors. Runners consume these while running. This is a relatively recent phenomenon, by the way. Only in the past couple of decades have runners begun to eat during runs themselves.*

moment but that they are capable of consuming a bowl of ice cream without fear or regret. Sometimes with whipped cream and sprinkles.

The Normal does his best to fill his shopping cart with fresh produce, whole grains, and that new high-protein strained yogurt from Finland that he keeps reading about, and usually he does, but those items are balanced with things like cream cheese and Cocoa Pebbles.

The Normal likes beer. A lot.

Coffee

Most adult runners, regardless of their subspecies and their dietary differences, are united in their love of coffee. In fact, for many runners, a cup or more of coffee before a run—especially a long one—has become a sort of ritual. For years, researchers struggled to understand why runners held coffee in such reverence. Did the brewing and drinking of the beverage have some ceremonial importance? Was it a way to fortify one's soul and awaken one's spirit before heading into "battle"? Or did runners drink coffee before a run just because it helps them poop?

The answer, as it turned out, is: All of the above.

Normals subsist on a diet of nuts, seeds, and berries. Also pizza. And burritos. And spring rolls, cheeseburgers, lo mein, chicken, various casseroles, shepherd's pie, stuffed mushrooms, fettuccine, tuna steaks, mashed potatoes, omelets, pancakes, waffles, gumbo, chili, cornbread, fish tacos, beet salad, eggplant Parmesan, breakfast cereal, yogurt, and whatever else you're offering.

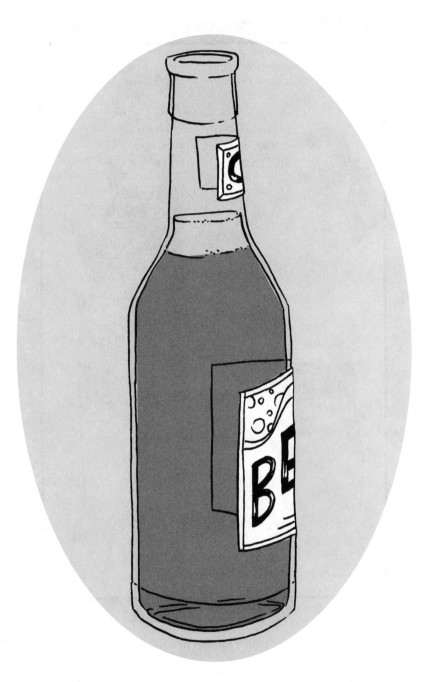

For many runners, the carbohydrate-rich liquid known as "beer" is a dietary staple.

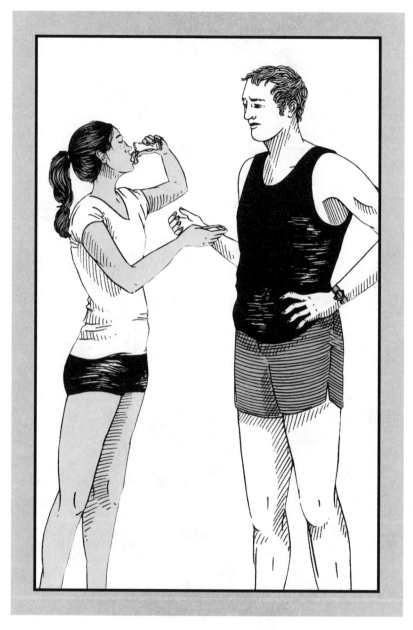

Runners share nourishment as a form of bonding.

The point is, Normals enjoy eating and aren't picky.

Will They Eat a McDonald's Hamburger?

BIRDS	An ENTIRE hamburger? Made of meat? Are you insane?
PURITANS	A FAST-FOOD hamburger? Are you insane?
NORMALS	Sure, and are you gonna finish those fries?

Notes

● Some runners, after a race that offers food, may be seen stuffing themselves with bananas and bagels and so on, carrying away as much as their mouths and arms can hold. We aren't sure what motivates this behavior, though some speculate that it may be an evolutionary drive to store food for the winter.

● You might be tempted to feed runners—especially the skinny ones—but don't do it. You'll only attract more of them, and runners swarming in great numbers can be a nuisance.

● If you must offer a runner food, never give it to him by hand. Though they are typically mild mannered, some runners may bite when frightened or excited (e.g., at the sight of a doughnut). Instead, place the food on the ground and slowly back away. Soon enough the curious runner will approach, sniff out the treat, and carry it away to be eaten.

● Due to a mild genetic defect, some runners have trouble understanding the abstract concept of the "calorie"; others are incapable of doing simple math without a calculator. Some runners suffer from both conditions. This can lead to trouble at meal and snack time—say, at a restaurant, when a runner uses that morning's 4-mile run to justify ordering something "smothered" in gravy.

DID YOU KNOW?

When unable to run for more than a day or two, many runners become visibly agitated; after a week, they may begin to pace their enclosure and gnaw on their own limbs.

CHAPTER 4

PHYSIOLOGY
AND
PSYCHOLOGY

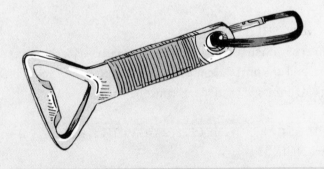

AS DESCRIBED AT LENGTH ELSEWHERE in this book, runners come in all shapes and sizes. For more on the particulars of a certain subspecies' physiology, please refer to the entry on the subspecies in question. The same goes for psychology, motivation, and so on.

This chapter is intended to provide a general overview of characteristics shared by all, or at least most, runners. Let's begin with a few basic questions and answers.

Physiology

WHAT KIND OF ANIMAL IS THE RUNNER?
Runners are mammals, meaning they have warm blood and nurse their young, though not while running. Males are typically larger than females. And more sensitive to pain.

SO RUNNERS ARE COVERED IN HAIR OR FUR?
Yes. For males, this can make removing Band-Aids from the nipples problematic. It also can present problems in very warm weather—as temperatures rise, the hairier the male the hotter it feels. Very hairy male runners are therefore the ones most likely to remove their shirts. They are also the males that you least want to see shirtless.

DO RUNNERS "SHED"?
In a manner of speaking, yes. Once or more per year—depending on the subspecies and amount of disposable income—runners will molt, discarding their old running shoes and replacing them with new ones.

DO RUNNERS CARRY THEIR OFFSPRING WITH THEM WHILE RUNNING?
Many do. Once their babies have developed necks strong enough to support their heads and skin thick enough to endure taunts such as "Run, Forrest, run!" from total strangers, runners may take them along for runs in wheeled devices called "jogging strollers."

NOTES ON GROOMING, HYGIENE, AND PREENING

● Despite their smell, most runners are quite clean, bathing daily or even more frequently, depending on when they run.

● Most runners also keep their bodies lubricated by applying petroleum-based substances to underarms, thighs, and genitals.

● Many runners—male ones in particular—will devote a surprising amount of time to developing firm muscles in the arms, shoulders, and abdomen. They will call this "upper body work" or "core work." In reality it is nothing more than a sort of preening, meant to attract potential mates.

● Runners spend an inordinate amount of time dealing with mucus—generating it, expelling it from various orifices, wiping it from hand to shorts and back to hand, etc. This puzzles researchers, who still aren't sure what purpose it serves. (With one exception: Hitting a fellow runner with snot, saliva, or phlegm may be seen as an act of aggression, or as a way to stake out one's territory while running.)

● Even very germophobic runners may willingly share food and drink with a fellow runner, but only while running. In one well-known move, one runner may drink from a fellow runner's water bottle—pretending that by holding the nozzle above his open mouth, he is somehow avoiding "germs."

● Certain runners—notably the Serious Runner, the Serial Marathoner, and the Ultra Runner—routinely take "ice baths." Despite their name, ice baths have nothing to do with hygiene. Scientists believe that sitting in ice baths may signal an early form of mental illness peculiar to runners.

● Most runners urinate—and, more rarely, defecate—indiscriminately and without shame. Trees, bushes, fields, vehicles … nearly anything can provide adequate shelter for a runner who has to "go," if the urge is strong enough.

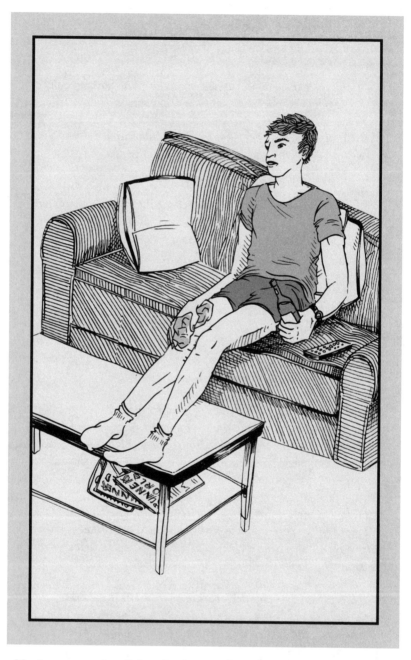

Most runners, when injured, return to the safety of their dens
to nurse their wounds.

ARE ALL RUNNERS DEAF?

No. This is a myth. It is true, however, that many runners over the past 15 years or so have sprouted small growths, or "buds," in or around their earlobes. These nodules make it difficult for them to hear, so you may have to shout to get their attention, warn them of danger, etc.

HOW HAVE RUNNERS ADAPTED TO VERY COLD CLIMATES?

Runners have evolved to puff themselves up in cold weather, adding layers to protect against the chill. Typically these layers are made of merino wool or synthetic materials designed to block wind and water while allowing moisture to escape.

ARE RUNNERS, ON AVERAGE, STRONGER THAN HUMANS?

No. Just more stubborn.

Psychology

Runners have many of the same emotions that we do. Runners can feel happy, sad, angry, afraid . . . sometimes all during the same race. Contrary to earlier thinking, runners *can* feel pain as well. Keep this in mind the next time you're tempted to throw an empty Snapple bottle at a runner from your car window.

Much like certain birds, runners have a fascination with shiny things. The promise of a cheap medal dangling from a ribbon will motivate some runners to endure hours of discomfort and even pain. This puzzles researchers, who have not been able to replicate the behavior in clinical settings, offering runners a medal for, say, walking barefoot on glass or jumping up and down for an hour.

IS THE RUNNER'S BRAIN SIMILAR TO A HUMAN BRAIN?

The runner's brain is very similar to a human's—it has two hemispheres and a six-layered cerebral cortex, for one thing, and looks really cool and gross all at the same time. There are a few notable differences, however. First and foremost, it is smaller, owing to the thickness of the runner's skull.

Second, a human brain plays a vital role in recognizing and processing pain signals, then deciding what to do about it; a runner's brain does not.

To understand this rather alarming distinction, let's imagine the following scenario:

Two specimens—a human and a runner—both in good health and of roughly equal weight, height, education, and socioeconomic status, stand side by side on the starting line of a standard-size running track. A gun fires, and both run quite hard for two laps, or 800 meters. (That's nearly half a mile.) By the time they finish, their legs are burning, their hearts pounding. They gasp for breath. Both are in a great deal of pain.

How their brains respond to this pain, however, is telling.

The human thinks to himself, "I am in a great deal of pain. To hell with this." And he walks away, in search of a cool drink and someplace to sit down. The runner thinks, "I am in a great deal of pain. But only five more to go, then I can do my cooldown." Then he runs five more 800-meter repeats, with 400 meters of jogging in between, and jogs a mile for his cooldown.

ARE RUNNERS INTELLIGENT?

This is an area of intense debate among human researchers.[1] On one hand, most runners exhibit clear signs of intelligence—they can recognize patterns, use crude tools, and know where to find online "promo codes" and apply them toward purchases of new running shoes. They even communicate with one another in their own primitive "language." (See Chapter 5, Language and Communication.)

On the other hand, runners often confound researchers with what seems a profound *lack* of intelligence. To use just one example, a runner may train for 6 months or more for a marathon; have an awful time during the marathon itself, emerging with debilitating pain, black toenails, and bloody nipples . . . and then register for another marathon almost immediately.

This apparent inability to learn—i.e., to use past experiences to inform future decisions—is a compelling argument against runners' being intelligent creatures.

---

1 *"Researchers who are human," not "researchers who study humans." You know what I mean.*

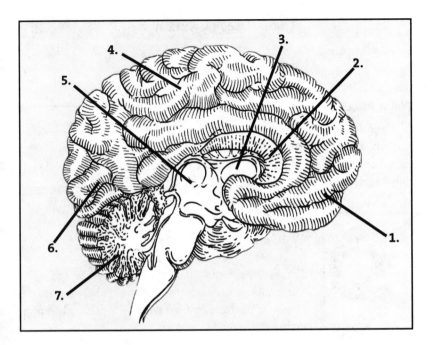

THE RUNNER'S BRAIN

Open the skull of a runner and you'll see a very familiar-looking brain.
You'll also be arrested and thrown into jail. So, please, do not open the skull
of a runner. Instead, let us give you a virtual peek.

1. "Pre" Frontal Cortex—aids in remembering and revering the late, great
Steve Prefontaine

2. Gore-Tex™ Cortex—creates desire for yet another running jacket even
though the brain's owner already has several perfectly good ones

3. Jitter Lobe—generates prerace jitters

4. Food Lobe—motivates in the procurement, preparation, and ingestion of
food in all of its various forms

5. Primary Motor Cortex—maintains forward motion even when other
parts of the brain protest

6. Painful Memory Suppression Gland—generates chemical substances
that diminish bad memories of the runner's last marathon

7. Everything Else—helps the runner think, breathe, etc.

Tools Used by Runners

Like many intelligent animals, runners are known to use tools—for grooming, defense, eating and drinking, and so on. Here are just a few.

FOAM ROLLER

Runners lie on and rub against these firm, often brightly colored cylinders—most often with their legs. Researchers aren't sure why but speculate it may be part of a mating ritual.

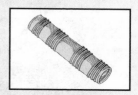

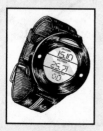

WATCH

It's the rare runner who's seen out and about without a watch. Most use them to measure their runs, in time or distance, or to record their "splits" during a workout or race. Others are thought to wear them solely to cultivate stark tan lines on their wrists—considered among some to be a sign of virility.

HYDRATION PACK

Runners use these backpack-style bladders to provide liquid, via a hose and mouthpiece, while running. The invention of hydration packs was a milestone for runners, who previously were forced to carry water or sports drinks in a handheld bottle during runs. Or to get slightly thirsty and wait a bit for a drink.

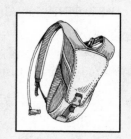

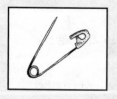

SAFETY PIN

This simple tool is used primarily in a prerace ritual wherein the runner opens the pin, carefully passes it through a bib number and shirt, and then jabs it into his or her chest.

ADHESIVE BANDAGE

Runners have appropriated Band-Aids and similar adhesive strips, using them not for scrapes and cuts but to guard against nipple chafing. They may also be used after a prerace safety pin ritual.

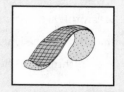

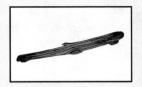

STICK

Scientists in the field often report seeing runners use sticks to pry small stones and other debris from the soles of their shoes. Or, more rarely, to jam small stones or other debris into the soles of their competitors' shoes.

CROSS-COUNTRY SPIKES

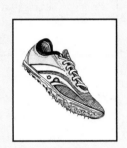

These thin, lightweight racing shoes are rarely seen. Used specifically for sloppy, muddy cross-country events, they employ rubber or metal spikes for better traction. This makes them impractical for everyday use, especially if you work someplace that has really nice floors.

Note that even runners who have never run a XC race in their life, and never will, are drawn to cross-country spikes simply because they're so cool-looking.

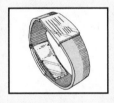

IDENTIFICATION BRACELET

Not to be confused with the tags used by scientists to track and monitor other animals, the runner's ID bracelet is intended to aid in the event of a medical emergency. Or for use after especially brutal marathons, if the wearer is unable to remember his or her name or address.

TRASH BAG

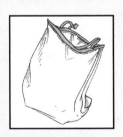

Exhibiting an ingenuity rare in most primates, runners have been known to use large trash bags for protection from the elements, fashioning them into crude "ponchos" and discarding them when no longer needed.

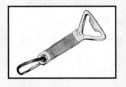

BOTTLE OPENER

This simple lever, which grants access to beer, is perhaps the runner's favorite tool. Most runners are never far from at least one bottle opener.

Q&A

Q: *My wife recently befriended a runner, who invited us to dinner. When we got a tour of her home, we were stunned at the number of running shoes she owned. My wife estimates she saw at least 20 pairs; I say it was closer to 30. Thirty pairs of running shoes! Is this normal?* —**Denny, Park City, Utah**

A: *It's not* abnormal, *Denny. Many runners hoard odd objects, such as shoes. Particularly when their favorite model is about to be discontinued. From an evolutionary point of view this isn't unusual—many species "stockpile" in anticipation of scarcity.*

ARE RUNNERS SELF-AWARE?

Yes. Runners are *intensely* self-aware. For proof, watch a runner who sees his reflection in a mirror. Especially a full-length mirror, and especially "in the wild," as he is running. Typical reactions include multiple sidelong glances—known as "checking one's self out"—with special attention paid to checking out one's calves and one's belly, or lack thereof.

WHAT MOTIVATES A RUNNER TO RUN?

This is a huge question, and as we describe in Chapter 2, runners run for a multitude of reasons. There is no single motivation. That said, in field surveys, a few themes do emerge. Here are a few of the most commonly cited reasons that runners run:

- Health and fitness
- Stress reduction
- Camaraderie (including the drinking that may follow the running)
- A sense of accomplishment
- Weight loss or management

It is popular among some humans to suggest that runners—especially those who run most (e.g., the Serious Runner, the Serial Marathoner, or the Ultra Runner)—are "running away from something" or are otherwise emotionally or mentally damaged. Researchers have found nothing to support this thesis and indeed have pointed out that nearly all humans have something worth "running away from" and very possibly would be happier and better adjusted if they spent some time running themselves.

DO RUNNERS SHARE A COMMON TEMPERAMENT?

To a certain degree, yes. Most runners are timid by nature. When approached, they will run away.[2] Over time, you can earn their trust. With patience and perseverance, you might even persuade a runner to let you touch him.

On a related note: While runners may all look alike to the layperson, they each have their own personalities, just like humans do. It is important to remember this when watching them in the wild. It is doubly important to remember when interacting with them.

ARE RUNNERS AWARE OF THEIR OWN MORTALITY?
DO THEY BELIEVE IN GOD?

Judging by how often you see them running with traffic, at night, wearing all black and with no reflective strips or lights . . . it would appear that no, many runners are not aware of their own mortality or indeed of the fragility of life. (This also adds to the case against runners being intelligent; see "Are Runners Intelligent?" on page 96.) As for a belief in God: Yes, runners as a group do tend to believe in God. More precisely, they believe in gods. Which gods they believe in will vary, depending on the subspecies. For example, for the Trail Runner, it is Kilian Jornet; for the Barefoot Runner, Christopher McDougall; for the Serious Runner, Jack Daniels; and so on.

---

2 *Come to think of it, maybe that's just them running. Whatever. Look, the point is that runners are timid.*

DID YOU KNOW?

Many runners are able to communicate with motorists using just one finger!

CHAPTER 5

LANGUAGE
AND
COMMUNICATION

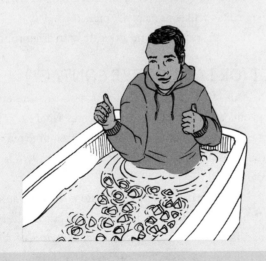

LIKE ANY ANIMAL, THE RUNNER must communicate to survive. Sometimes this takes the form of a shriek and a gesture made to an oncoming motorist. Sometimes it means raising an outstretched hand to someone offering cups of water. Other times it is much more subtle; even a runner's body language can "communicate" a wealth of information, if you know how to interpret it. And in many cases, yes, runner communication involves actual speech.

In this chapter, we'll explore two kinds of runner communication: runner-to-runner and runner-to-human.

Runner-to-Runner Communication

Regardless of subspecies, ethnic background, or geographical location, all runners speak the same language—i.e., Runglish,[1] a curious blend of English, metric, and the Swedish word *fartlek*, spoken and written in a manner that nonrunners find perplexing. The only exception to this is the Newbie, whose command of Runglish is (yes!) tentative. As the Newbie's running skills develop, so too will her grasp of Runglish.

Here are some of the ways runners communicate with other runners.

EYE CONTACT (OR LACK OF EYE CONTACT)

For reasons researchers are still struggling to understand, two runners passing each other in opposite directions will sometimes avoid eye contact. Even if there is no one else around. Or one runner will attempt to make eye contact—usually in a friendly way, in an attempt to "connect"—while the other studiously avoids it.

Is this a tacit display of dominance and submission? No one is sure.

In any event, it is hardly universal. In many other instances, the scenario plays out much differently, with both runners making eye contact, exchanging some sort of greeting (usually a very subtle one), then continuing on their ways.

---

1 *If you're wondering whether this makes it okay to refer to runners as Runglishmen, the answer is yes.*

BUMPER STICKERS

The most obvious of these bear such messages as RUNNER, RUNNER GIRL, or I ❤ RUNNING. (Actually, such slogans appear to be intended not for fellow runners but for humans.) Other bumper stickers may say things like "26.2," a reference to the marathon distance; "13.1," the half-marathon; or even "0.0," which means that the runner who owns that car likes to "have fun with it."

Other stickers are so cryptic that only certain fellow runners will understand them—e.g.,

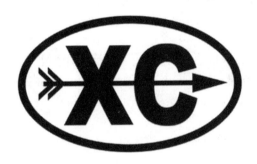

("Cross-country")

SOCIAL MEDIA

Communication on social media platforms, most notably Facebook, may take the form of long conversations. More often, they look like this:

> **RUNNER 1's status update:** "Ran 5.8 miles."
>
> **RUNNERS 2–12:** [LIKE]

Note that even on social media, runners can quickly sniff out an impostor in their midst. Usually when someone mentions a "5-K marathon."

HAND SIGNALS

Humans will find many runner hand signals familiar—from the simple upraised-palm "hello" to the simple upraised-palm "good-bye," which are actually the exact same hand signal, which is not as confusing as it sounds.

When running in packs, runners might literally point out hazards in the road, such as potholes, cracks, roadkill, etc., to runners behind them.

When angered, runners may raise a single middle finger. This tells the recipient, "You have displeased me. Please reconsider your actions. Good day to you, sir."

During a race, a runner who is suffering especially badly may express his state of mind to onlookers by clutching his throat with both hands and sticking out his tongue.[2]

During a race, a runner who passes a spectator blowing cigarette smoke across the course may express his state of mind by clutching the spectator's throat with both hands. Or just glaring.

POSTURE AND FACIAL EXPRESSION

A runner's posture can say a lot about his physical condition and/or state of mind. A tall, erect posture says, "I am aroused" and "Tights were a poor choice today."

A hunched upper body says, "I am tired"; a hunched lower body says, "I am *really* tired."

A horizontal body says, "I have finished" or "I cannot go another step" or both.

A doubled-over, hands-on-knees posture says, "I am vomiting or am about to vomit."

A runner's arms are reliable indicators of exhaustion. A loose, relaxed arm swing, front to back, means all is good. Conversely, a short and jerky arm swing is usually bad news. A runner seen "shaking out" her arms means that she is consciously trying to remain loose and relaxed. A runner seen "shaking out" another runner's arms means that she is not well and probably needs medical attention.

Likewise, facial expressions may convey any number of emotions, from pain to amusement. A runner may exhibit any number of these, just in a single race.

---

2 *This author has direct experience with this, as proved by a photo taken of him around mile 22 of the Boston Marathon, circa 1998.*

A MARATHON, IN FACIAL EXPRESSIONS

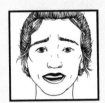

Prerace:
Nervousness

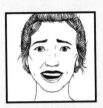

Start:
Euphoria

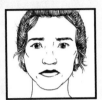

Mile 5:
Mild boredom

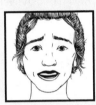

Mile 10:
Nervousness

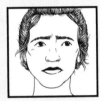

Mile 16:
Doubt

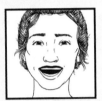

Mile 20:
Happiness

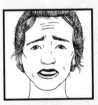

Mile 21:
Terror

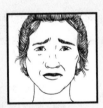

Mile 23:
Pain

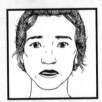

Mile 24:
Oblivion

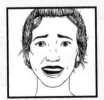

Mile 26:
Euphoria

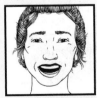

Finish:
Orgasmic joy

Postrace:
Pain

A runner who is limping badly, in obvious distress, may have recently finished a marathon. With their limited mobility, such runners are easy targets for predators; it is estimated that as many as 15 percent of recent marathon finishers are overtaken and killed by lions, bears, and other meat eaters.[3]

Human-to-Runner Communication

Most North American runners speak English or Spanish passably well. They can ask for directions to the nearest restroom, for instance, or order food in a restaurant—although runners who have just completed a marathon or ultra may manage only to point at the menu and grunt.

IS THAT RUNNER A JERK?

You greet a passing runner, and he doesn't respond. Is he a jerk? It depends . . .

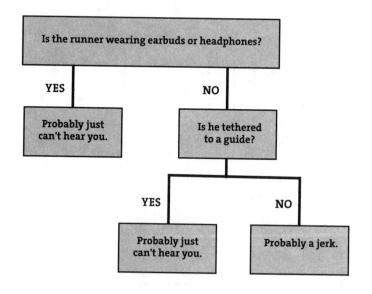

---

3 Source: *Running USA*

The appendix in the back of this book will help you speak with runners about running—or at least understand what it is they're talking about. But what if you want to have a "real" conversation with a runner? What if you want to talk about something other than running?

It can be done, with patience and practice. Just be aware of two things:

1. A skilled runner will find a way to steer almost any topic back to running. For example,

TOPIC OF CONVERSATION	RUNNER'S CONTRIBUTION
"My dad had hip surgery last week and is recovering really well."	"Speaking of hip surgery: Did you know it's a myth that running is bad for your joints?"
"How about this weather, huh?"	"Tell me about it! I ran 10 miles this morning, and it was unbearable."
"Man, [Politician X] is a real piece of work."	"You got that right. Hey, did you know he ran a 4:35 marathon a few years back?"
"So, what do you do for a living?"	"I'm a [white collar job title]. Which is lucky for me, because I run SO MUCH, I can't imagine having a physical job on top of that."
"I'm so sorry for your loss. Your mother was a wonderful woman."	"Are you going to finish that lasagna? I ran long this morning and I am *starving*."

Watch for signs of this happening so you can rein things in while you still can.

2. Much like a Wi-Fi signal, a runner's attention span weakens the farther it gets from its source. Go far enough and it's lost completely.

Put plainly, a runner is most attentive and engaged in a conversation when the topic is running. The further you stray from that, the more stunted your conversation will be.

The visual on the following page may help you.

THE RUNNER'S CONVERSATION TARGET

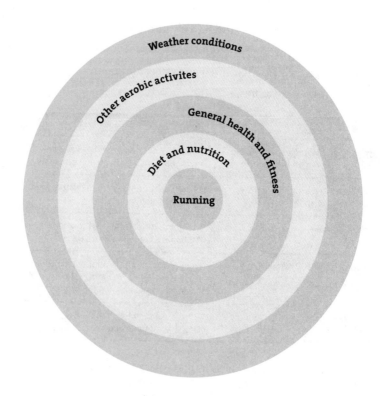

Out of Bounds

*Politics, religion, arts and
entertainment, pop culture,
current events, history, etc.*

By using simple words and learning a few key Runglish phrases, you can
carry on a simple conversation with a runner for as many as 5 to 10 minutes.

Q&A

Q: *I live near a runner who has been training for a marathon. When I saw him recently, he looked terrible—he was skinny, his cheeks were sunken, and his eyes seemed hollow. When I asked if he was sick, he perked right up. Has he lost his mind?* —Paul, Austin, Texas

A: *This is a terrific way to illustrate the language barrier between runners and humans. When you suggested he looked "sick," your friend—who sounds like a Serious Runner—took it as a compliment. Serious Runners know they're ready for a marathon when their appearance frightens humans.*

DID YOU KNOW?

The technical term for a group of runners is a "group."

CHAPTER 6

SOCIAL BEHAVIOR AND MATING HABITS

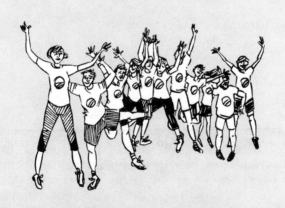

AS WE HAVE SEEN TIME AND AGAIN in this book, runners as a population are hard to classify. This difficulty extends to their social and group behavior, which can be surprisingly complex—certain runners prefer to run alone, while others can't stand solitude. Still others, perhaps the majority, are ambi-social, enjoying both kinds of running. These runners may run alone, with one or two close friends, or in a large group, depending on their moods, schedules, and so on.

Interpersonal behavior among runners—both between and within subspecies—is similarly sophisticated and may be influenced by any number of factors.

The mating habits of runners, on the other hand, are really very simple. Much like humans, runners just want to have sex. As often as possible. Preferably but not necessarily with someone of their own subspecies.

But we're getting ahead of ourselves! Let's first take a closer look at social behavior.

Runners: Social Animals, Sort Of

It was once thought that runners spent nearly all of their waking time engaged in one of the following three activities:

- Preparing to run
- Running
- Recovering from a run

Q&A

Q: *I've overheard runners using the word "chick," but as a verb—e.g., "I got chicked at last weekend's 5-K." Is being "chicked" a good thing or a bad thing?*
—Peter, Akron, Ohio

A: *When a male runner says he was "chicked," it means that a woman caught and passed him during a race—especially in the final stretch. Almost always, this term is used in a good-natured way.*

With today's more advanced research techniques, we now know that runners devote significant time as well to these activities:

O Talking about preparing to run

O Talking about running

O Talking about recovering from a run

Nowadays, of course, "talking" is used loosely and can mean anything from tweeting to Instagramming to Facebooking. In rare cases, it can also mean "talking."

This is notable because it means that runners are more social than previously believed. As recently as 20 years ago, many researchers (and laypeople) encountered runners almost exclusively in situ—i.e., out running, often alone. Sometimes in rainstorms. As a result, it was believed that runners were not only solitary creatures but also insane. (As we noted in Chapter 4, most runners are *not* insane.)

> ### Social Hierarchies and Running Shorts
>
> *Does "shorts length" convey some unspoken message about social standing? Some scientists believe so. The length of one's shorts seems to carry a special significance, particularly for males. Some runners choose shorts that go nearly to the knees and practically billow in the breeze. Others prefer shorts that fall around midthigh. Still others—often, but not always, Serious Runners—opt for "short shorts," which can virtually disappear under an untucked shirt. A handful of highly aggressive males wear shorts that are so short we could not show them here without pixelation. This is widely seen as an act of hostility. If you see such a runner in the wild, give him a wide berth.*

Today, thanks to the explosion of the Internet and social media, it is painfully clear just how social runners can be.

Many social traits found among runners will look familiar to anyone who has studied animal behavior:

O In most communities of runners, you will find one alpha male. Typically he is a local guy who "ran D-1 in college" and has a half-marathon PR of 1:09 or better.

(continued on page 118)

The 7 Types of Runner Photos

Much like their human cousins, runners love taking and sharing photos of themselves. Virtually all of these photos fall into one of seven categories.

1. THE PRERUN SELFIE

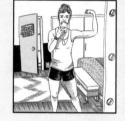

What is it? A photograph taken of the runner, by the runner, before he or she embarks on a run. Typically showing at least one outstretched arm. Facial expressions may range from happy and smiling to stone-faced.

What purpose does it serve? It is thought that the Prerun Selfie is used as a sort of advertisement for one's suitability as a mate.

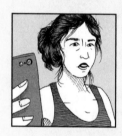

2. THE POSTRUN SELFIE

What is it? A photograph taken of the runner, by the runner, immediately after finishing a run. As in the Prerun Selfie, we see at least one outstretched arm holding the phone used to take the photo. In this version, however, the subject may appear tired and disheveled, and often glistens with sweat.

What purpose does it serve? Resembling as it does a postcoital snapshot, the Postrun Selfie is definitely used to advertise one's suitability as a mate. I mean, come on.

3. THE MIDRUN SELFIE

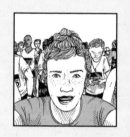

What is it? A photograph taken of the runner, by the runner, during a run.

What purpose does it serve? Researchers speculate that the Midrun Selfie is a "cry for help," as it telegraphs to viewers the subject's recklessness and disregard for her own well-being.

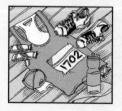

4. THE NIGHT-BEFORE-THE-RACE "FLAT RUNNER" PHOTO

What is it? A "still life"-style photo showing the clothes, shoes, and other gear that the subject intends to use for an upcoming race—typically one happening the next morning.

What purpose does it serve? Experts are divided. One theory is that the Flat Runner photo, which in a sense can be described as "a runner without the runner," is a manifestation of existential dread, serving to convey the subject's awareness of the ephemeral nature of life and her subconscious struggle to accept the knowledge that every one of us, ultimately, will vanish from this earth, becoming as invisible as the "runner" in the photo and to literally "keep moving forward" despite that knowledge.

Another theory is that runners just think running gear looks neat.

5. THE GROUP SHOT

What is it? A photograph taken of a group of runners, often before a run or race. Subjects may be wearing matching shirts.

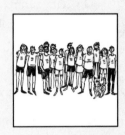

What purpose does it serve? The Group Shot serves to strengthen the social bonds among, and define the identity of, those belonging to the group. Also it's a chance for shorter runners to be in front.

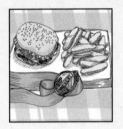

6. THE LOOK-AT-THIS-FOOD-I'M-ABOUT-TO-DEVOUR SHOT

What is it? A photo of foodstuffs—often but not always conspicuously "unhealthy"—that a runner is moments away from eating. Taken in many cases shortly after a long run or race, such as a marathon.

What purpose does it serve? Thought to be a vestige of the days that runners traveled in packs and would gather around a "kill" to eat side by side. As that practice is no longer feasible, or socially acceptable, this social media equivalent has emerged to take its place. (These photos almost always feature some sort of meat.)

7. THE ICE BATH SHOT

What is it? A photograph, usually taken by someone else, showing the subject sitting in a bathtub full of ice water after an especially hard or long run or race.

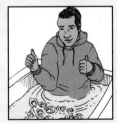

What purpose does it serve? This one is also a cry for help.

(continued from page 115)

O   Likewise, most regular groups of runners—even those organized only loosely—will have a "leader" that they follow. This leader will often act as a mentor for younger or newer runners in the group, organize long runs, dispense justice, and be the butt of good-natured jokes.

O   In running groups dominated by males, competition can be fierce for the attention of the few females.

O   Some runners can be very territorial, going so far as to claim a certain treadmill at the gym as their own.

O   Runners may be found interacting with other sports species, such as cyclists and triathletes. Usually such interactions are peaceful. But not always.

O   Rivalries with other groups are not uncommon. Most notably, runners and joggers have a history of tension and mutual distrust.

Courtship and Mating Habits

Little is known of the mating habits of runners, as attempts to observe and record them usually result in the subjects calling the cops. Here is what we do know:

For males, the courtship process begins gradually, perhaps with him inviting the desired female on a short run. After a period of acclimation, during which the male and female will talk, laugh, and get accustomed to each other's sweat, the male will "ratchet things up" with an invitation to dinner or a movie. Before they know it, the male is wearing a novelty T-shirt with a slogan such as "Distance Runners Do It Longer" and the female can resist him no longer.

At this point, hydration occurs—typically with beer, wine, or Long Island iced teas—followed by application of body lube, to reduce chafing.

The act of copulation begins slowly, as both parties warm up with light aerobic activity. Things then heat up. Through a series of ups and downs, including a few moments when they question whether they'll

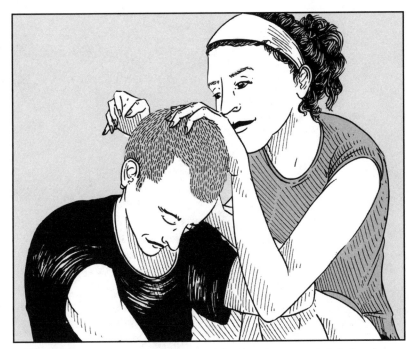

Like other primates, runners use social grooming to maintain hygiene and to reinforce social bonds.

ever finish, they persevere. In rare cases, one or both parties may cramp up, requiring a short break before resuming.

By the time they reach the finish line, they are hot, sweaty, exhausted—and euphoric. It was long and hard, but they did it!

Can humans and runners successfully breed?

Humans and runners certainly have their differences, most notably in temperament and in number of race shirts deemed acceptable to have lying around. But their "plumbing" is the same. This is important, because incompatible plumbing—especially in the bathroom—can cause all sorts of problems. Relationships are difficult enough without having to deal with burst pipes, leaks, and inoperable drains.

So, yes. Humans and runners can—and do!—breed. Society hasn't always approved of such unions. But, thankfully, times have changed. Today it is not unusual to see a human and a runner "out and about," playing, shopping, and dining just like any other couple—often with children in tow.

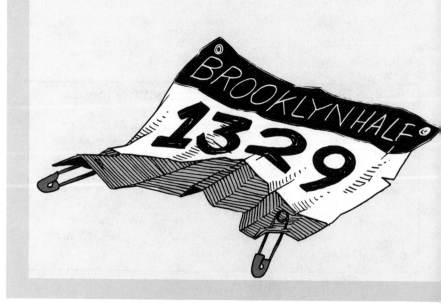

PART III

DID YOU KNOW?

When they dress in real clothes, some runners
can easily pass as human. Perhaps you see runners
every day and don't even know it!

CHAPTER 7

LIVING AMONG
RUNNERS

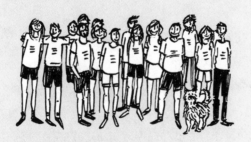

AS WE NOTED IN CHAPTER 1, the number of runners in recent decades has exploded. For the runners themselves, this has been a blessing and a curse. On one hand, it's never been easier for a runner to find a race of just about any distance. Running gear is better than ever. And runners are judged a lot less harshly than they used to be.

On the other hand, there is only so much "habitat" out there. With humans developing more and more land, runners are forced onto streets and roads, suburbs and cities. As a result, encounters between runners and humans have risen sharply. Usually they're harmless. But at times these interactions can cause tension, anxiety, and unease.

This chapter is meant to help you minimize such unpleasantness in your own dealings with runners in various settings.

Are Runners Dangerous?

You should never provoke them, of course. But runners by their nature are docile and will go out of their way to avoid confrontation. However, females pushing jogging strollers may attack if they feel their babies are in danger. Also, hearing certain phrases might enrage runners; among them:

- *"Running will ruin your knees."*
- *"Marathons cause heart attacks."*
- *"Hey, you're a jogger, right?"*
- *"Jogging will ruin your knees."*

Runners who hear any of these may respond forcefully. Meaning, they will go on Facebook and complain.

Note that "jogger" comments can be especially provocative, depending on the mood of the runner in question and/or how tightly wound he is to begin with. Calling a runner a "jogger" is almost always considered a grave insult and may inspire violence. Particularly if it leads to an exchange like this one:

Runner: "Do I look like a jogger?"
You: "Yes."

On the Road

The runner's biggest threat, by far, is the automobile. Please keep this in mind when you get behind the wheel! Give runners as much room as you can, slow when passing, and refrain from honking—even if you mean well, it can startle an already nervous runner.

Outside Your Home

If you grow vegetables or have fruit-bearing trees, you may wake some Saturday or Sunday morning to find a group of hungry runners helping themselves during a break in their long run. If this annoys you, it's easy enough to discourage. Loud noises frighten most runners, so banging on a pot or shouting will likely send them scampering away. You may be tempted to install a scarecrow-style mannequin to frighten runners away. Don't. Such gimmicks usually backfire, as they actually wind up attracting runners wanting to take selfies with the scarecrow.

Runners may not be *that* bright, but they're smarter than crows.

Inside Your Home

Especially in the hot summer months, runners may seek relief in air-conditioned homes and then panic when they can't get back out—especially once they realize that their GPS watch has lost its satellite connection. If you discover a runner stuck in your home, open a door and try to shoo her out with a broom. If that doesn't work, try a little trickery. Pointing outside and shouting, "Hey! Isn't that the guy who wrote *Once a Runner*?" has been known to work.

At a Party, a Bar, Etc.

From time to time, a runner may stray from his pack and find himself in unfamiliar territory, such as a sports bar or a dinner party full of extroverts. Often he will appear agitated or confused.

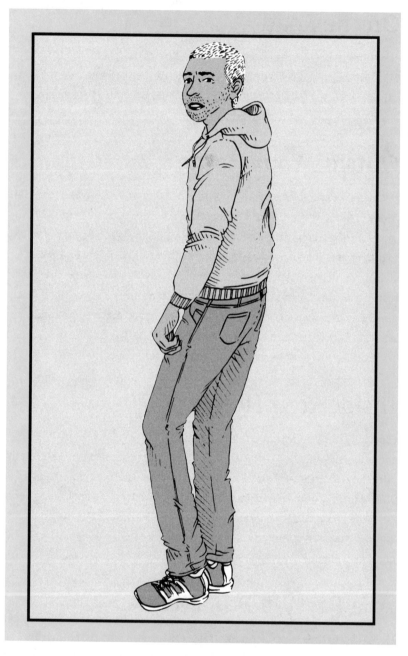

Dressed in normal clothing, many runners can—and do—
pass as human.

Don't panic! Runners can sense anxiety, and it will only make a bad situation worse. Instead, approach the runner and ask about his footwear or his watch. Both will likely be running-specific. Soon he will be talking about running nonstop, which will put him at ease. This will buy you some time while someone phones the nearest specialty running store. The store will send someone to collect the runner and return him to safety.

Q&A

Q: *More than once I have seen a runner who appears to be chasing a dog. Sometimes it looks like the runner has already lassoed the dog and is attempting to rein him in. Do these runners intend to capture and eat these dogs? If so, that is awful.* —Peter, St. Louis, Missouri

A: *No! Rest assured, the runners you saw had no intention of harming those dogs, much less killing and eating them. Much like their human counterparts, runners long ago domesticated animals, such as dogs, for companionship and affection. Many of these "pets" even accompany their owners during runs. This is what you're witnessing.*

DID YOU KNOW?

If you stand very still, with a cup of water in your outstretched hand, you can get a runner to come right up to you. This works best if you are standing near a marathon race course.

CHAPTER 8

STUDYING AND OBSERVING RUNNERS

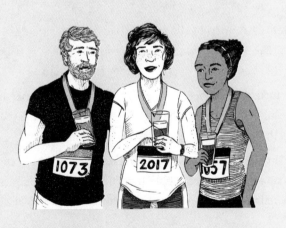

RUNNER-WATCHING CAN BE AN EXCITING and rewarding hobby, if you're patient. It offers all the excitement of bird-watching—if you can believe that!—with the added advantage of not being pooped on by the subjects you're watching.[1]

They may all look alike at first, but over time you will be able to distinguish among any of several subspecies—even perhaps among individual runners within the same subspecies.

Many communities now have runner-watching clubs that meet to spot runners, identify their subspecies, and discuss their shared fascination with runners.

Here are several tips and general principles to keep in mind when you set out to study runners:

○ Maintain a calm, quiet demeanor. Even strong, confident runners will go out of their way to avoid confrontation or other potentially unpleasant encounters.

○ If you're a smoker, wait until later to light up. Runners of all kinds find cigarette smoke repellent and will do just about anything to avoid or escape it.

○ Conversely, runners of all kinds find certain other scents irresistible—brand-new running shoes, for instance. Rub a pair over your body before heading into the field.

○ You can also try attracting runners by imitating a runner distress call (e.g., by shouting, "GAH! My calf!") or by playing the theme to *Rocky* through a portable stereo.

○ Note that while watching runners is perfectly fine, trapping them is no longer socially acceptable. In fact, many municipalities have outlawed the practice—even when "humane" traps are used.

---

1 *However, remember that runners are primates, and like certain other primates they may fling poop if they feel especially agitated. For this reason it is recommended that you wear old clothing while observing runners in the field. And eye protection.*

How Can I Attract Runners to My Yard?

It's fun and easy to make your yard into a runner-friendly zone, encouraging more of these creatures to venture close. There's nothing quite like looking out of your kitchen window in the early hours of the morning and seeing a group of runners in your very own backyard!

Here are some tips for turning your property into a haven for runners.

- Hang friendly signs, flags, etc. on and around your home (e.g., WELCOME FRIENDS doormat; happy pineapple banner; WE ♥ RUNNERS flag). Avoid signs reading "This Property Protected by Smith & Wesson."

- Plant fruit trees for runners to graze on and tall bushes on the perimeter of your property. Runners often urinate behind tall bushes.

- Keep your dogs penned or inside the house. Especially if their names are Smith and Wesson.

- Adorn the cars in your driveway with "26.2" bumper stickers.

- Have a garden hose out and in plain view. Especially on hot days, runners seek out water.

- Smear pinecones with peanut butter and hang them from low tree branches. Few runners can resist free peanut butter.

- Leave a trail of "energy bars" from the nearest road onto your property. Don't worry about other creatures eating them; they will be repelled by the smell and taste.

- If you have the resources, runner decoys are an excellent way to attract runners. A few used department store mannequins dressed in running gear should do the trick. Arrange them around your property. For added effect, have one "urinating" into a bush.

What Equipment Do I Need?

Not much. A good pair of binoculars can help. Comfortable clothing—nothing too flashy—and a sturdy pair of shoes. (You may have to do a bit of running yourself.) A notebook for recording your findings. Mostly, you need perseverance—runners are notoriously wary creatures!

It's easier to get close to a runner who is wearing earbuds or headphones. But be warned that these same runners will startle easily once they're aware of your presence.

Where to Find Runners

For aspiring runner-watchers, bringing the runners to your home is one approach. But it's hardly the only one. No matter where you are geographically, runners tend to congregate in any of several common locations, where they can be observed safely and easily.

PUBLIC PARKS

Public parks are natural attractions for runners. However, they attract plenty of other species as well. For this reason, consider visiting a park when the weather is poor or in the early morning. This may sound unappealing, and in some ways it surely is. But it is actually a terrific way to spot runners. Humans, including those who may be dressed as runners, tend to stay home when the weather turns very cold, hot, or wet; actual runners do not. Hence, nasty weather has a filtering effect, eliminating visual clutter for those seeking to spot runners.

RUNNING TRACKS

If you're wanting to get a good look at a certain type of runner, a public running track is a surefire bet. High schools are a good place to start, assuming they allow the public to use their tracks during off hours. (Call to find out.)

Interestingly, the two basic kinds of runners you can expect to find at a track are virtual opposites—the Serious Runner, on one hand, and the "I'm Not a Real Runner" Runner or the Dramatic Weight Loss Runner on the other.

They are drawn to the track for different reasons. The Serious Runner goes to do speed work, i.e., timed, fast repeats of 200, 400, 800 meters, and so on; the "I'm Not a Real Runner" Runner or the Dramatic Weight Loss Runner will show up just to log a mile or three in relative peace and quiet and away from traffic. Look for the Serious Runner in lanes one or two and the others in the track's outside lanes, near the walkers.

SPECIALTY RUNNING STORES

Most towns or cities of any size will have these retail outlets, which cater to local runners of all kinds, offering shoes, apparel, and other gear. Many specialty running stores[2] also offer clinics, group runs, and other events, acting not only as a shop but also as a social hub.

These stores therefore offer an excellent, and reliable, way to see runners up close in a safe environment. If you're nervous about interacting with runners, you can simply view them through the store's windows. Don't tap or knock on the glass; this can disturb or frighten the runners inside.

WARNING!

You may try to get "up close and personal" with runners by posing as one yourself. This can work for a time, but note that you will almost certainly be found out if you try to talk about running. Especially if you try to pronounce Keflezighi. Worse, if you do fool the runners, you risk being pulled along into an actual run. Possibly a very long one.

---

2 *If you're seeking actual runners, and not just humans shopping for running shoes, be sure to visit an independent specialty running store and not a national footwear chain—even if it advertises itself as an "authority" on "sports."*

(Continued on page 136)

Photographing Runners

As we've noted throughout this book, runners by nature are timid creatures. However, in the presence of a camera they become outgoing and even hammy. Especially in groups. This is known as the Pentax Paradox, named after the man who first noted and wrote about it, Steve Pentax.

To see this paradox in action, head to your nearest running path—or, better yet, a local race—and stake out a good vantage point with your camera. As a group of runners approaches, raise your camera, call out, and watch them transform from a fairly serious and quiet bunch into a collection of exhibitionists. Some of them may raise their arms and shout, "WOOOO!"

This appears to be a reflexive, involuntary response, and it can be a useful thing; professional race photographers, for instance, take full advantage of it.

The one notable exception to this phenomenon is the Trail Runner. As noted earlier (see pages 70–71), Trail Runners are skittish and very distrustful of humans.[3] The presence of a camera only intensifies this response. Those wishing to photograph Trail Runners might consider using a tree stand, such as the ones used by deer hunters, or constructing a blind.

A Trail Runner blind needn't be elaborate or even very sophisticated; you can use whatever materials you have on hand. Something as simple as a large cardboard box will do. Just cut a small flap or slot around eye level, place it near a trail known to be popular among Trail Runners, sit inside, and wait. Sooner or later, if you're lucky, your patience will pay off.

Note: Do try to position your blind upwind from the trail. While Trail Runners have poor-to-average sight and hearing, their sense of smell is quite keen. Especially if you have food.

---

3 Humans are the ones who are destroying nature!

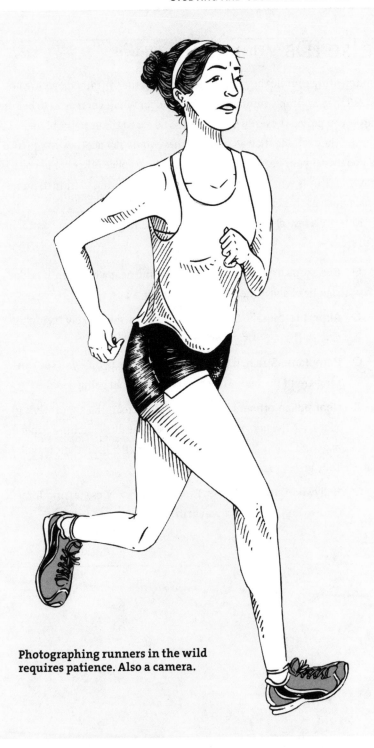

Photographing runners in the wild requires patience. Also a camera.

False IDs

Some creatures, while they look like runners to the untrained eye, are not. Instead they're simply humans who happen for whatever reason to be running. If you pulled these "runners" aside and asked them, point blank, whether they self-identify as runners, they would say no. They might also tell you to "get your hands off" them or call for a police officer or pepper-spray you. This is why it is best to leave this sort of thing to trained professionals, such as this author.

Here are a few places where runner misidentification most commonly occurs.

- **Bus stops.** If you see someone running near a bus stop, it is likely that he or she is merely trying to catch a bus.

- **Airport terminals.** Likewise, except he or she is likely trying to catch a flight with a tight connection.

- **Pamplona, Spain.** If you also see bulls, the people you see running aren't runners. They are trying to avoid being gored.

- **Near police officers.** That naked guy screaming about "flying saucers"? The person in the ski mask? The duo clutching paper bags and leaving a trail of fluttering small bills in their wake? They aren't running. They are fleeing.

- **Hollywood movie shoots.** Especially for movies starring Tom Cruise. Tom Cruise is always running in movies.

The Footwear Fallacy

Amateurs are often fooled into thinking they can spot a runner by his or her shoes. Don't fall into this trap. Counterintuitive as it may sound, the presence of running shoes is NOT a reliable way to identify a runner in the field. Humans have adopted running shoes as their casual footwear of choice and wear them everywhere from the supermarket to traffic court. Sometimes they call them sneakers.

Note that if you see a 40-something-to-60-something-year-old man wearing cotton socks with a specific style of running shoe—sturdy, white leather, made by New Balance—you have identified not a runner but a subspecies of human called the Middle-Aged Suburban Dad. These creatures are mostly harmless.

DID YOU KNOW?

*If they continue reproducing at today's rate,
runners could become North America's
dominant species by 2050.*

ENDNOTE: TRENDS AND PREDICTIONS

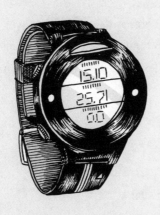

AS RECENTLY AS THE 1950S, there were fewer than 50,000 runners in North America. Thanks to improvements in diet and shoe technology, and to magazines like *Runner's World*, it is estimated that that number today has swelled to 65 million.[1]

This proliferation is good news for manufacturers of technical apparel and the artificial dyes found in sports drink flavors with names like "Orange," but it raises serious questions about the planet's finite resources and how they're allocated. How many servers must be added to handle the millions of social media posts published every day by runners sharing details of their latest run or photos of their new shoes? How many square miles of COOLMAX® can be worn before dangerous levels of moisture are wicked into the atmosphere?

And for how long can the planet afford to feed millions of runners? The sport bean plantations of Central and South America, which produce 90 percent of the world's sport beans, are tremendous consumers of resources. One pound of sport beans takes as much as 28 gallons of water to produce, much of which is used for irrigation.

For these reasons and more, runner colonies on the moon or on Mars are being seriously discussed.

It also means that humans and runners must learn to coexist in a more gentle, symbiotic manner. Now that you understand runners a little bit better, it is my hope that we all can work together to make this happen.

Go in peace!

---

1 *Margin of error: +/- 50 million.*

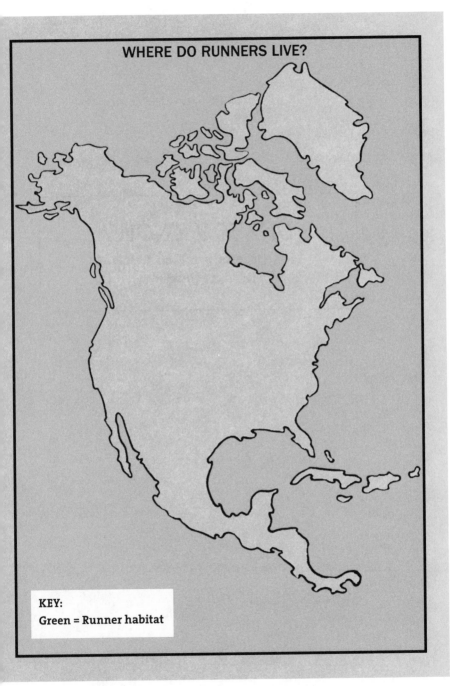

DID YOU KNOW?

*Runners have appendixes,
just like humans do!*

APPENDIX

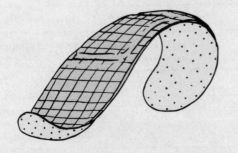

Runner-to-English Translations

Speaking with runners can be daunting. In addition to their own jargon and specialized terms, they also use everyday English words to which they have assigned new, and sometimes baffling, meanings. This glossary will cover the basics.

WHEN A RUNNER SAYS...	YOU MAY *THINK* HE MEANS...	BUT HE REALLY MEANS...
bandit	masked villain in a Western	someone who runs a race without paying for it
bib	the thing that babies wear while eating	the thing that runners wear while running—a sheet of plasticized paper displaying a number unique to that runner
bonk	the act of hitting one's noggin, e.g., on a low ceiling, branch, etc.	to suddenly and catastrophically run out of energy, especially during a long run or race
chick	a baby chicken or a female human (mildly offensive)	the act of a female runner passing a male runner during a race (mildly offensive, sometimes, to the male being passed)
DNF	that band in the '90s?	Did Not Finish, as a race
fluids	any liquid (with possibly R-rated connotations)	water and sports drinks
fuel	gasoline	food
healthy	in good health	intact; without apparent injury; able to run without (too much) pain
jogger	one who jogs	someone overly slow or not serious about running; often derogatory

WHEN A RUNNER SAYS...	YOU MAY *THINK* HE MEANS...	BUT HE REALLY MEANS...
'k	okay; sure thing; yes	kilometer
minimal	the least amount possible	running shoes with little to no "support"
negative	less than zero; bad; "no"	running the second half of a run or race faster than the first
positive	more than zero; good; "yes"	running the second half of a run or race slower than the first
PB	peanut butter	personal best
PR	public relations	personal record
repeat	"huh?"; "come again?"; "I didn't catch that"	a segment of predetermined time or distance, run at a predetermined pace
speed	velocity	a speed workout (see "workout")
split	share; depart; cut in half	a runner's time over a precise portion of a run, race, or workout
taper	a slender candle	a period of relative rest and recovery before a race, usually lasting 2 or 3 weeks
tempo	speed, especially of a piece of music	speed, especially the kind that makes you want to cry because there are no breaks
wall	a vertical structure that separates two adjacent spaces	an invisible structure that you "hit" when your body depletes its energy supplies
workout	something involving free weights, probably at a gym	something involving repeats (see "repeats") or hard continuous effort

The Runners of North America Checklist

While out in the wild, be it urban or rural, keep your eyes peeled for each of the runner subspecies described in this book and check them off this handy list. Feel free to add in any additional information and tell your friends on social media!

SUBSPECIES	LOCATION	NOTES
THE NEWBIE ❑ Male ❑ Female Date Spotted: / /		
THE "I'M NOT A REAL RUNNER" RUNNER ❑ Male ❑ Female Date Spotted: / /		
THE CLUB RUNNER ❑ Male ❑ Female Date Spotted: / /		
THE FITNESS RUNNER ❑ Male ❑ Female Date Spotted: / /		
THE BUCKET LISTER ❑ Male ❑ Female Date Spotted: / /		
THE WEIRDO RUNNER ❑ Male ❑ Female Date Spotted: / /		
THE FASHION MAG RUNNER ❑ Male ❑ Female Date Spotted: / /		
THE SERIOUS RUNNER ❑ Male ❑ Female Date Spotted: / /		
THE ELITE RUNNER ❑ Male ❑ Female Date Spotted: / /		
THE HIGH-INTENSITY CROSS-TRAINER ❑ Male ❑ Female Date Spotted: / /		

SUBSPECIES	LOCATION	NOTES
THE ADVENTURE RACER ❑ Male ❑ Female Date Spotted: / /		
THE DRAMATIC WEIGHT LOSS RUNNER ❑ Male ❑ Female Date Spotted: / /		
THE BAREFOOT RUNNER ❑ Male ❑ Female Date Spotted: / /		
THE MOM RUNNER ❑ Male ❑ Female Date Spotted: / /		
THE DAD RUNNER ❑ Male ❑ Female Date Spotted: / /		
THE GRIZZLED VET ❑ Male ❑ Female Date Spotted: / /		
THE 7:00-MINUTE-MILE GUY ❑ Male ❑ Female Date Spotted: / /		
THE GEAR ADDICT ❑ Male ❑ Female Date Spotted: / /		
THE CHARITY RUNNER ❑ Male ❑ Female Date Spotted: / /		
THE SERIAL MARATHONER ❑ Male ❑ Female Date Spotted: / /		
THE TRAIL RUNNER ❑ Male ❑ Female Date Spotted: / /		
THE ULTRA RUNNER ❑ Male ❑ Female Date Spotted: / /		
THE KID RUNNER ❑ Male ❑ Female Date Spotted: / /		

FOR FURTHER READING

There are many fine books and publications devoted to runners and running. To learn more, visit your local library or bookstore or go online and check out these resources.

WEB SITES

runnersworld.com

BOOKS

The Runner's Rule Book, by Mark Remy (Rodale, 2009)
The Runner's Field Manual, by Mark Remy (Rodale, 2010)
C Is for Chafing, by Mark Remy (2011)

PERIODICALS

Runner's World